gentlebirth

Your
Positive
Birth
Begins Here

The ultimate guide to a positive empowering pregnancy
and birth experience - as defined by YOU!

TRACY DONEGAN

Tracy Donegan is a Midwife, author and Founder of GentleBirth. Tracy is the mother of two gorgeous boys and better half to her life partner and business partner Philip. Passionate about empowering parents to have the best birth possible, Tracy provides support information and inspiration to parents around the world preparing for a positive birth. Tracy currently lives in California.

CONTENTS

INTRODUCTION

*"You do a lot of growing up when you're pregnant.
It's suddenly like, Yikes. Here it is, folks.
Playtime is over."*
–Connie Fioretto–

Have these thoughts crossed your mind during your pregnancy?

What if there's something wrong with my baby?

What if I poop/puke/scream/cry in labor?

Are my breasts the right size to breastfeed?

What if I'm not a good mom?

If any or all of these thoughts have crossed your mind and you've found yourself suddenly in a cold sweat (not hormone related) then this book is for you. Between these pages is the power to radically change how you think about pregnancy, birth and parenting. And how you think about these things changes the way you experience them.

So let's do this!

Here you are – pregnant...possibly terrified, and probably overwhelmed with the books, baby stuff and let's not forget the buckets of unsolicited advice from the pregnancy police. Let me start off by saying how very humbled I am that you have chosen my book to help you prepare for one of the biggest (if not THE biggest) transitions of your adult life. (Yep you're officially an adult now). In your hands you're holding the equivalent of Harry Potter's Book of Spells – except this isn't about magic – it's about mind, medicine and midwifery. But first lets address the elephant in the room - this is not a book about natural birth – my greatest wish for you is to have a positive experience - however you define that to be. That could be an epidural in the parking lot or swinging from the chandeliers a la Sia.

GentleBirth is more of a mindset than a method. My approach of tried and tested techniques and exercises will challenge and change the way you think and shift your mindset incredibly quickly so you can savor this time even more and have a healthier more enjoyable postpartum period with your new baby (your partner will thank you too).

I'm a midwife and a mother and am here to support you through this transition. So, although you may have been recommended my book to prepare for your baby's birth, I want you to know that so much of what you're going to learn will help you long after your baby arrives. I've taken a brain science approach to pregnancy wellbeing, birth preparation, and parenting. It's such an exciting time to be a midwife and to have an opportunity to share this information with you.

As with all of the brain training in this book, if you find any practice emotionally challenging, give yourself permission to take a break for a few days and begin again or talk to your care provider.

THE MOST IMPORTANT JOB IN THE WORLD

Take a moment to imagine you are an alien who has just arrived on planet earth and you are pregnant *(this new world of pregnancy and parenting often feels alien to almost every first-time mom)*.

On planet earth, we tell women all the time that being a mother is the most important job they will ever do (and it's true). You are about to take on the role of a lifetime. You are about to experience profound changes in your body, your mind and your heart...it will change everything about you – how you see yourself, how the world sees you and how you see the world. If you were this alien you would start to realize how important you are and how life changing this next chapter of your life would be.

Knowing this you would probably be very keen to find out what you can do to prepare for such an important job. What training do you need to succeed and where do you get this important training? What skills can you learn in the coming months to make this transition as empowering and as positive as possible?

On planet earth preparing new mothers for the role of a lifetime doesn't match up to the importance of this life-changing event in a woman's life that we keep telling her about. If this pregnant alien went to a bookstore what would she find? (Inspiration doesn't seem to make it to these shelves very often).

It's likely that she would find a lot of books that focus on everything that can go wrong during this time. On TV she would see more scary stories... What would other women tell her? They'd probably tell you how terrible birth is...and how difficult being a new mom is. Newfound friends might direct you to YouTube to watch videos that leave you terrified. Your care provider might even direct you to a class with other parents for 8 hours of training in diaper changing, baby bathing, the signs of labor and how your partner can massage you. These are all helpful to know but the skills of resilience, focus and the ability to mother in a way that is self-compassionate and nurturing (the skills that really matter for the 'role of a lifetime/ most important job on the planet') are nowhere to be found.

Wouldn't that pregnant alien feel very confused - aren't you? We keep insisting that this is the most important job in the world but the preparation we offer mothers is minimal and often focused on what's wrong instead of what's right.

If this alien decided to become an accountant consider how much training and preparation they would have (4-year college degree plus about 20 hours of exams and countless hours of exam prep).

If being a mom is the most important job in the world then we need to up our game.

What if that alien had new training available to her, if she had the ability to prepare for birth - and life after birth with tools and training that inspired, uplifted and excited her about the changes ahead?

Starting around 12 weeks that mom would have completed several thousand hours of preparation just using the GentleBirth App. Best of all most of that preparation is done at home...on the couch or in bed for about 20 minutes each day. You could also attend a live class with your partner of an additional 12 hours and ongoing support from your Instructor and a global community of well prepared new moms. We've made it easy to prepare for the most important job ever - and enjoyable too!

What if that preparation left you feeling confident and reassured that even with these great changes and great challenges of motherhood - also comes great joy.

"You had the power all along my dear"
–Glinda the Good Witch–

Words have power and the stories you tell yourself about birth and parenting impact your pregnancy and your body during labor and birth. Will your beliefs and thoughts about yourself make your baby's birth and parenting experience more manageable or more challenging? Every woman has the potential to have a positive birth experience but some of us need more convincing or we don't believe we are deserving enough. Think about whether you might be getting in the way of your positive birth and how you can change that. That potential for great births is in all of us but it's been hidden away, buried deep under layers and layers of misinformation, dramatic TV shows, and fear. I'm going to help you to uncover the innate wisdom every mother has - that "knowing" that there has to be a better way, a more gentle way. You already know how to grow your baby; it's part of your genetic makeup. Let's face it as human beings we're pretty good at birth (we continue to overpopulate the planet each year). My intention is to remind you of something you have long forgotten, a rediscovery of your power. Today you can begin immersing yourself in the new science of positive, healthy, powerful, and gentle birth. Day by day your thinking will begin shift and your body will begin to respond to the anticipation of the birth process rather than the fear of it. You begin to act as if a positive birth isn't just possible - it's probable. I'll be with you every step of the way and next to you as you bring your baby into the world. The voice in your ear telling you that "you can do it" will be so much louder than the voice in your head telling you that you can't. You've got this.

THE GENTLEBIRTH APP

Reading this book is a great start to a more enjoyable pregnancy and birth but to take your birth preparation to the next level download the GentleBirth App (available in the App Store or Google Play with a free trial). Depending on your unique journey the GentleBirth App will guide you in your daily practice and support you in any twists and turns you may have to navigate. Come meet our growing community of GentleBirth moms around the world in the GentleBirth official private Facebook group - a sanctuary created to inspire, uplift and excite you during your pregnancy. For readers who prefer a more hands-on experience and plan to take our immersive classes, you'll find a list of GentleBirth Instructors at http://www.GentleBirth.com

BIRTH STORY

The Perfect Birth

I thought I should get around to sharing my GentleBirth story before I forget too many details! My actual birth experience was better than I had ever envisioned my 'perfect birth' could be. I had an atypical experience; my doula and the hospital nurses had never seen anything like it. I'm so thankful to the GentleBirth community for helping me grow and welcome our daughter into our family! (sorry this birth story is quite verbose)

I attended a GentleBirth workshop early (at 5 months), since I would be travelling, and am so glad I attended when I did! I started the hypnosis and mindfulness training immediately. It took me many months to be comfortable doing them without any tracks and also became part of my daily routine. It also helped me stay positive through my pregnancy, when the ultrasounds kept saying she was small for her size (she was born perfectly normal!).

I started my maternity leave 5 days prior to my due date (Oct 17) and was feeling wonderful. I was confident and excited to introduce our first child into the world. I had a doula that I'd talk to constantly and loved. She helped me create an all-natural birth plan that I rehearsed in my head many times (which included spending the majority of labor at home, then rushing to hospital to give birth in under an hour). I had a hospital bag packed with Wonder Woman socks and sports bra, yoga pants and snacks for the nurses. I also had a gift bag of goodies I put together for my husband after the birth.

Twice during my 39th week, I had 12 hours of prodromal labor throughout evenings. They would start around 10pm and intensify throughout the night, then fizzle out the next morning. I even called my doula and midwife convinced I was in labor at 3am once! These surges were some of the worst I experienced throughout this journey, but I was able to use deep breathing techniques and counter pressure to get through them with a smile. At 39 w 6 d, my midwife said I was dilated 4 cm and guessed I would give birth within the next few days (I was thankful the prodromal labor was doing something). At 40w 6d, my midwife swept my membranes (without asking, and just told me that she "stirred things up"), but I just took this as something I couldn't control and accepted it. At 41 wk, I had another episode of prodromal labor; this one starting in the afternoon. This time, I put on pop music and danced with my husband through every surge and we had a ton of fun. In between surges, we watched movies and got most of the way through a Where's Waldo book. The next day, I was laying on the couch, watching Twilight (guilty pleasure), and I thought my water may have broken, so I called my midwife's office. The nurse told me she didn't think I had, since I wasn't having any pain or surges, but she'd tell the doctor anyway. To keep my mind occupied that night, my husband and I went out shopping and ate delicious Mexican food. When returning home, the doctor called and suggested that I go into the Birthing Center and get checked, just to be safe. I arrive around 7pm and the midwife on call said I was between 6 and 7 cm and said that she could see hair (I wasn't leaving the hospital). She was shocked that I was still smiling and not in any pain (other then minor back ache).

Decked out in my Wonder Woman attire, I watched football with family, walked laps around the halls with my doula and had a dance party with my husband and doula through intermittent surges. At 3am, I was at 9.5 cm and still smiling and walking the hallways. The nursing station was shocked and amused every time I'd pass, smile and wave. I hadn't changed at all when the midwife re-checked at 7am, right before shift change and mentioned that the next midwife might suggest augmentation, since I wasn't progressing or having normally spaced surges. She was right and this initially terrified me! My husband and my doula kept reminding me to stay positive and I was placed on Pitocin at 10am. The nurse increased my Pitocin dose quite quickly, and soon I was having 5 min long surges with little to no rest in between. At 2pm (19 hrs at the hospital), I was exhausted from all the dancing and pain and was given a pain reliever through the IV (Nubian). I was so thankful for a few minutes of respite! An hour later I was able to start pushing and at 41.3 weeks at 4:24pm my beautiful baby girl was born at 8 lbs.

▍THE MISSING LINK

As you've no doubt noticed from your lustrous locks and developing cankles your body undergoes incredible physiological changes in pregnancy, so it seems reasonable that your brain undergoes significant changes too. All joking aside pregnancy changes your brain but not in the ways that your favorite sitcom would have you believe. Very few birth professionals have been taught about this complex "engine" (your brain) that controls your pregnancy, birth, and breastfeeding experience. Don't believe me, ask your OB or midwife about brain plasticity in pregnancy and be prepared for an uncomfortable silence and probably some awkward paper shuffling. Over the last decade, there has been an increased focus on comfort measures for labor - water birth, doulas, peanut balls but all of these happen when pain already exists - essentially after the horse has bolted when you're IN pain. By learning how you can sculpt, remodel, and retrain your brain to "think again" - you can change those pain signals and how your brain interprets them. After your baby arrives your 'mommy brain' will, in fact, help you be more sensitive and responsive to your newborn baby – your brain is being sculpted for survival of the species.

Recent studies indicate (contrary to the media reports) that your brain "upgrades" in pregnancy. During pregnancy and in the first hours after birth your brain has literally been reconstructed by hormones and by your interactions with your baby in the important hours after birth. Researchers Kinsley and Fransen describe these massive brain changes as being 'like the revving of a high-powered sports car at the starting line' getting ready for the starter's signal for the new demands of motherhood. Are you impressed yet? Although I will admit that some days I felt like my brain was far from firing on all cylinders. Pass this section to your partner so they can read this too. In pregnancy you're like the bionic woman– your brain is being rebuilt. No doubt you're well aware of the benefits of physical exercise. Training the brain brings additional improvements for health and wellbeing. Training your mind and sculpting your brain is not dissimilar to sculpting your biceps and, like any fitness-training program, it takes ongoing practice and daily commitment (but it's so much more enjoyable and it won't leave your hair frizzy). One trip to the gym or a walk in the park does not significantly improve your health daily practice with the App makes a difference. If you're wondering how you'll fit in all of this wellness training into an already busy schedule – you'll be happy to hear that the longer brain training sessions in the App can be done from the comfort of your couch or bed...and you'll enjoy deeper, more restorative sleep during your pregnancy (what a nice side effect)!

By reading this book, you're are taking a big step forward toward a positive, empowering, and more comfortable birth experience no matter what happens on the day and life skills that will stay with you forever as you parent more gently too. Each time you practice you're building emotional resilience - the ability to "bounce back" from setbacks and handle stressful situations in a healthier way. Resilience is the ability to face and handle life's day-to-day challenges with a flexible and adaptable attitude throughout your life.

Over the years, one of the most exciting aspects of my work isn't the increase in positive births (although it is so thrilling to hear those incredible birth stories). Where GentleBirth really shines is the ability for moms and partners to handle whatever comes their way on the day. In the event of a difficult birth experience, you have the tools and insights to reframe a negative birth experience into something more positive – these are important skills to develop for parenting and you won't find them in other birth preparation programs. You are developing and mastering incredible skills for birth and parenting and not just building yourself a better brain but you're changing how your baby's brain develops too. Your daily training will change the way you respond to the world forever. Learning how to not "sweat the small stuff" changes your life and your experience of it - as a mother and a parent.

You can use the App at any time during your pregnancy and experience the benefits of a more relaxed pregnancy and more positive mindset.

Throughout the book you'll see that I've focused on three core areas of birth preparation for the most positive birth possible:

1. Brain training.
2. Physical comfort measures & head hacking.
3. Negotiating the best birth for you (and your baby).

With the daily practice recommendations, you and your baby can enjoy the benefits of less anxiety and more excitement (more sleep is also a great 'side effect'). It's my wish that this book brings more joy to your pregnancy and more calm back to your baby's birth. You are joining thousands of other women all over the world who are choosing to rethink birth - calm, comfortable, and in control.

THE GENTLEBIRTH
IMPACT ON BIRTH OUTCOMES

Here's where things get really interesting. In 2014 a large research study of 34,000 women compared different nonpharmacologic (natural) pain management approaches to labor (Chaillet 2014). When compared with other nonpharmacologic approaches to pain, childbirth education that was based on intentionally activating specific parts of the brain is associated with a significant decrease of epidural analgesia, caesarean births, instrumental delivery, use of synthetic oxytocin, longer labors and lesser maternal satisfaction with childbirth. The results were so impressive that the Canadian Association of Obstetricians created a clinical guideline based on the results so that careproviders understand more about the biology of pain to provide more effective support in labor. This book and your daily app practice mirrors the research recommendations. So if an unmedicated birth is important to you, the GentleBirth approach lines up with the most improved birth outcomes by any childbirth education approach available today.

Dr. Christiane Northrup, obstetrician and author of Women's Bodies, Women's Wisdom, expresses it well in her book when she forwards a challenge to all birthing mothers:

"Imagine what might happen if the majority of women emerged from their labor beds with a renewed sense of the strength and power of their bodies, and of their capacity for ecstasy through giving birth.

"When enough women realize that birth is a time of great opportunity to get in touch with their true power, and when they are willing to assume responsibility for this, we will reclaim the power of birth and help move technology where it belongs--in the service of birthing women, not as their master."

BRAIN

I Cannot Wait for Labor!

"I cannot wait for labor. I'm not stupid, I know it can go in different directions to what I envisioned. But the one thing I absolutely know won't go in the wrong direction is my mindset. And to me that makes me a winner."– Leanne Keane (3 months before Leanne gave birth).

THE BIRTH OF LILLIE

My first two pregnancies, seven and five years ago, were very very different to this one. I was very overweight, extremely unfit and had zero confidence. Through changing enormously as a person since my third pregnancy and subsequent labor were very very different.

Due to a tragedy within my immediate family last year, I was anxious as my "due" date approached. Half of me wanted so badly to wait for a spontaneous labor and the other half wanted to get started ASAP and be done with all the worry and fear.

The day before my "due" date I had a minor meltdown with community midwife who sent me to the hospital for a full checkup and a chat with the doctor. Thankfully the doctor I saw was very understanding of my feelings and agreed to an induction the following Saturday at 40+4. I was instantly calm. I had no problem with being induced as it went so well previously (@ +14) and not once did I become nervous in the days that followed.

Saturday morning arrived as I got the last bits together and kiddies went off with my father in law. Even still I was perfectly calm and ready to set about the task ahead. We arrived in the hospital, did admissions, etc., and waited for the doctor. Upon examination at 9:30am, baby's head wasn't engaged and it was too risky to break waters so a 24-hour, slow-release propess was inserted instead. Within the first hour I was having cramps and by 2:30pm I was having contractions that could be timed. I walked the corridors with my fast playlist in, did squats, took 20 minutes rest, used the birthing stool (but found it very uncomfortable) and sat on my yoga ball. On the ball I rocked my hips, leaning on the bed with earphones in alternating with my music playlist and the 10-minute GentleBirth meditation. By 6pm, the contractions were less than 2 minutes apart so the propess needed to be removed. Once it was, the contractions got much stronger and, over the next two hours, I was full sure we were on the home front. I mostly stayed on the ball, put all my attention on my breathing and actually found myself using hand gestures similar to a wave in line with my breath. I was so happy with how well I was working through it all.

And then it stopped. By 8:30pm the contractions had basically disappeared. I had cramping in the hours after but nothing more. One of the community midwives came to see me at 11pm and advised me to get some sleep and see what the doc said in the morning. I won't lie, I was pretty upset. I had a little cry and off I went to sleep for 2 hours. (My dad owns an apartment 1km from hospital so my husband walked to it to get some sleep, safe in the knowledge he could be back in a flash if needed be). I woke at 1:30am and then got another one hour of sleep at some stage later.

Sunday morning my husband was back by 7am. We had breakfast and anxiously waited for the doc to arrive. My concern was that there would be no more they could do for me and I'd be sent home and back to square one with the worry I had all along. Thankfully, the 6 hours work put in yesterday had brought baby's head down low enough that my waters could be broken. I was thrilled.

Once done, I was totally back in the game. Not much happened throughout the day, my parents came to see us and my mam ended up staying seven hours with myself and husband in the ward. We relaxed and chatted and ate and laughed with the sun shining in the window as we waited for my body to do its thing. By 8pm that night I was pretty shattered and fell asleep only to be woken an hour later with the first of the "official" contractions at 9pm. No mistaken this, things were kicking off.

Labor and Birth:

9pm-11pm was pretty ok. Within 30 minutes I had my TENS machine on as I knew this was it. By 11:30pm, contractions were 2-3 minutes apart so I asked to be checked. Not quite far enough along to go to the delivery room. Community midwife gave me two heat packs, one for tummy, one for lower back, put my GentleBirth back on (Labor Companion and affirmations) and lay on my left side with husband doing hip compressions during each contraction. I feel I coped quite well throughout but by 1am was eager to get to delivery. 1:10am and it was time to go.

Arrived in room 9 where my daughter had been born 5 years earlier, I was delighted it was available. We got settled in setting up my fan, my phone with speaker and the wireless trace was put on. I leaned on the bed (which the midwife had raised up) and swayed my hips. I used the gas and air, did squats on the exhale and spent a lot of time with my eyes closed. The first few tries of the gas and air I felt dizzy but I quickly realized I just needed to focus on my breath AFTER each contraction ended and the dizziness passed. We chatted in between contractions about my playlist and the singers on it. I smiled as I spoke of how my mam used to sing the song playing, "The Greatest Love of All" by Whitney Houston.

After some time I asked to use the shower. I LOVED it on my last labor. At this stage, it was 2:30am or thereabouts (as per my labor notes). I didn't get to stay long as the trace kept moving. I also hit a bit of a wall and felt exhausted. I got out of the shower and lay on the bed but couldn't relax nor get comfortable. I tried the right side, all fours and leaning over the back. But I'd lost my flow. I asked for Pethidine—it was the turning point.

Once administered, I actually began to lightly snooze in between contractions. When I felt one starting I'd put gas and air back in and when it passed I'd nod off slightly. Getting those few minutes each time totally rejuvenated me and gave me the energy I needed to continue.

Some may find the rest of my story bonkers, some may resonate. But it was an experience that could only be felt. It's for this reason it has taken me so long to try to put it into words as I simply don't know if I can, but here goes.

My head and my mind left the room. I went into the deepest state of relaxation I've ever experienced. I asked for silence in the room to allow me to stay where I had gone. My husband and midwife kindly obliged. I spent the next long while leaning over the back of the bed, TENS now gone, gas and air in hand. I was unaware of what was going on in the room. I could feel my body moving and swaying and rocking when I realized I wasn't controlling it. There was no longer "pain" during the contractions. It was like as if, when each one began, a sensation changed in my body but it stayed at the one level. And then it went away again.

While I was unaware of my immediate surroundings, I heard another mother in labor being very vocal. I just remember thinking it was like an animal noise. I could resonate with her. I could sense her. I felt she helped me and I helped her. If I did have any moments of doubt during this time, once I heard her vocalize I instantly felt "we're in this together". The word I used to describe this whole experience to my dad later that day was primal. I felt a bit silly at first but that's just how it felt. Like I was experiencing what animals do when they give birth—in fact, how it should be for humans also.

By around 5:30am, my body started making sudden movements. It was almost like something was inside me and trying to get out—which is literally what was happening. I later read in my notes the phrase "expulsive contractions" and that's exactly how it felt. It was my body signaling it was ready to deliver my baby. There was no need for examination to check I was 10cm, it was extremely clear.

I became aware there were now more people in the room. The midwife had made a call just to let others know we were about to deliver should she need assistance (my daughter was 9.14 lb. and had slight shoulder dystocia). I recall turning back around from leaning over the back of the bed, pulling my legs back and reaching down and feeling my daughter's head. I couldn't believe it; I genuinely hadn't felt a thing. No burning or stinging sensation she had literally slid out. Inside that same contraction, with a bit of a push,

Lillie Grace Keane was on my chest. At the very last moment, I got a bit lost. I remember squeezing my husband's hand but not knowing where I was for those few seconds (it was almost like coming around from being really dizzy). And then almost like somebody waking you from your sleep, I was back in the room.

I remember looking out the window and wondering how it was bright, it was morning, 5:55am with the most beautiful red sky.

Lillie lay on my chest under my nightdress and didn't get dressed until the next day. She stayed in her nappy on my chest only coming out for feeds and a nappy change. Once we got to the ward she latched on first go not a bother. 8 weeks later I can't say it's been an easy road with all sorts of problems but the main thing is we're still breastfeeding and making progress. Having only lasted 1 day with Dylan and Ava I'm over the moon and absolutely loving it. The feeling you get when feeding, for me, is like the icing on the cake after a wonderful birth-something you would struggle to put into words—and I get to feel it all day every day.

GentleBirth brought me back to neutral. Anytime throughout my pregnancy, my labor, my delivery that I drifted, it brought me back to where I needed to be. In the final days of my pregnancy when anxious I adjusted one affirmation to "I stay with my baby in these last few days". Repeatedly in delivery, I reminded myself out loud, "soft body strong mind". The 10-minute meditation was a Godsend when I was stressed in pregnancy. And the induction track helped me refocus what exactly induction is; just a different starting point.

Our baby is here, 8 weeks old today, we are all in love and I am so so so thankful for the wonderful and beautiful experience that I finally got to see, that birth really is.

TELLING A NEW BIRTH STORY

"In giving birth to our babies, we may find that we give birth to new possibilities within ourselves."
–Myla and Jon Kabat-Zinn–

Don't Hook Your Happiness on One Kind of Birth

I'm not going to tell you that your birth will be pain free, easy or short and if anyone does run the other way. For most first time moms your labor experience will fall somewhere in the middle but there are things that you can do to stack the odds in your favor of it being less painful, a little easier and maybe even shorter. For years we only had two choices in how we planned to cope with labor - pain-free with medication or medication-free and in pain. But there's no reason why you can't enjoy a more positive and gentle birth no matter how your baby arrives on the day – that's why mindset matters so much. Our philosophy has always been that a positive birth comes in many forms and is defined by you – not friends, family, or the nosy neighbor down the street. But what's equally important is that you have a gentle emotional experience of pregnancy, birth and the postpartum period. This is a time for self-compassion and self-kindness. I invite you to allow GentleBirth to provide you with a raft of buoyancy as you navigate the sometimes stormy seas that are ahead.

Let's get down to basics. You didn't have to learn how to digest your food and you probably never took a class on how to pump your heart. By using the practices in this book you're reducing fear of birth and replacing it with confidence, you're going to learn how to tune out distractions and tune in to your natural instinct. It's about turning off the negative thought patterns and turning on the primal, instinctual part of the brain that makes birth a more positive experience. It all sounds complicated but, in reality, it's very simple. In fact, it's the simplicity of GentleBirth that makes it seem too easy. The same part of your brain that controls digestion, your breathing, your eyes blinking, making sure just the perfect amount of blood gets to every nerve muscle and fiber in your body is the same part of the mind that is responsible for reproduction and birth.

The same part of your brain that developed and released the perfect egg (for most readers) and created the exact conditions for a healthy pregnancy - is the same part of your mind that is responsible for the unique hormonal dance between mother and baby that starts labor and helps birth 'happen' – without any conscious input from you. Most moms are able to work, drive, and attend to life's day-to-day demands without consciously thinking about how to grow their baby. You just trusted that your body knew what to do, where to put your baby's eyes, ears, fingers, and toes. You didn't wake up one morning and think to yourself, "I need to grow my baby some ears today." So, after nine months of pregnancy, do our amazing bodies just "forget" how to get the baby out? Of course not.

Your body has incredible potential but in birth just like in life sometimes we can be blindsided by an unexpected turn of events or an illness and there are times when our body can do some strange things. Most books prepare you for the birth you want – I want to take things one step further to prepare you for the birth you didn't want.

"Remember this, for it is as true as true gets: Your body is not a lemon. You are not a machine. The Creator is not a careless mechanic. Human female bodies have the same potential to give birth well as aardvarks, lions, rhinoceri, elephants, moose, and water buffalo. Even if it has not been your habit throughout your life so far, I recommend that you learn to think positively about your body."
–Ina May Gaskin–

GENTLEBIRTH THROUGH THE AGES

As early as the 1800s, scientists were discovering that women who didn't expect birth to be a traumatic ordeal tended to have more comfortable and shorter labors.

Here is an excerpt from "Labor among Primitive Peoples" by George Julius Engelmann, written in 1882:

Two or three years ago (1879-1880), an Indian party of Flat Heads and Kootenais men, women, and children, set out for a hunting trip. On a severely cold winter's day, one of the women, allowing the party to proceed, dismounted from her horse, spread an old buffalo robe upon the snow and gave birth to a child which was immediately followed by the placenta. Having attended to everything as well as the circumstances permitted, she wrapped up the young one in a blanket, mounted her horse, and overtook the party before they had noticed her absence.

Dr. Grantly Dick-Read tells us about a birth he attended that changed his own perception of birth: "In due course, the baby was born. There was no fuss or noise.

"Everything seemed to have been carried out according to an ordered plan.

"There was only one slight dissension: I tried to persuade my patient to let me put the mask over her face and give her some chloroform when the head appeared and the dilation of the passages was obvious.

"She, however, resented the suggestion and firmly but kindly refused to take this help. It was the first time in my short experience that I had ever been refused when offering chloroform. As I was about to leave some time later, I asked her why it was that she would not use the mask. She did not answer at once, but looked from the old woman who had been assisting to the window through which was bursting the first light of dawn: It didn't hurt. It wasn't meant to, was it doctor?"

Long before his time, Read made the connection between fear and the expectation of excessive pain in labor.

"For far too many, pregnancy and birth is still something that happens to them rather than something they set out consciously and joyfully to do themselves"
–Sheila Kitzinger–

GENTLEBIRTH IN MODERN TIMES

In more recent times, obstetrician Dr. Michel Odent has been helping the world rediscover the needs of the birthing mother and what he refers to as "undisturbed birth." According to Dr. Odent, we must focus on the most active part of your physiology in birth - the brain and the glands orchestrating the perfect hormonal release to make birth more manageable. The same hormones that were present when creating your baby (for most moms) are the same hormones needed to birth your baby: dim lighting, privacy, and the freedom to be yourself. In order for your hormones to work optimally during labor, certain conditions need to be met, such as a quiet, relaxed, comfortable atmosphere where you feel safe and supported and have privacy. Believe it or not, the hormones of romance are also the keys to great labors (more on that later).

You've been practicing (yes practicing) the thoughts of fearful birth and excessive pain for a long time so you're probably really good at it! Like any bad habit, we can change it, and once you change those beliefs your life will never be the same again. TV shows like "One Born Every Minute" and even reading lots of dramatic birth stories weaken your neuronal network for positive birth. GentleBirth reconfigures your brain for emotional wellbeing and a positive birth.

▌WHAT ABOUT DADS?

Becoming a parent is one of the biggest life transitions we go through and, as moms, we're living the experience but dads (life partners) are spectators and in our current society – quite uncomfortable ones and often forgotten when it comes to paternal postpartum depression. Research suggests that 10% of new dads experience paternal postpartum depression.

We're only starting to get to grips with the stigma associated with mental wellbeing in pregnancy for moms. It's so important to keep this conversation going to raise awareness but we need to widen the circle of support to include dads/partners. The stigma against experiencing difficulties in early parenthood is even higher for men than for women. We expect them to be stoic, strong and selfless... but when a new dad is having difficulties they're even less likely to ask for help. Dads and female birth partners have their own brain training within the GentleBirth App.

YOUR MINDSET MATTERS

Harvard psychologist Professor Ellen Langer has spent her entire career investigating the power of the mind. Langer's research started over 30 years ago, in 1979, when she carried out a ground-breaking study. She wanted to know whether recreating a state of mind from 20 years earlier would make any changes in the bodies of participants. A group of elderly men in their late 70s or 80s were recruited for a "week of reminiscence." Surrounded by props from the 50s they were asked to act as if it was actually 1959. They watched films, listened to music and discussed news events of the time - all as if these things were new and happening right in the present.

Understandably, Dr. Langer herself had doubts. "You have to understand, when these people came to see if they could be in the study and they were walking down the hall to get to my office, they looked like they were on their last legs, so much so that I said to my students, Why are we doing this? It's too risky."

As the week went by Dr. Langer began to notice that they were walking faster and their confidence had improved. One man decided to do without his walking stick. At the end of the week, they played an impromptu game of touch football.

Physiological measurements were taken both before and after the week and showed that the men improved across the board. Their gait, dexterity, arthritis, speed of movement, cognitive abilities, and memory were all measurably improved. Their blood pressure improved and, even more surprisingly, their eyesight and hearing got better. The subjects' joints became more flexible, their posture straightened, and the lengths of their fingers, which typically shorten with age and arthritis, increased.

In another example of Langer's research, she took 84 hotel housekeeping staff and told one group of them that the work they did (cleaning hotel rooms) was good exercise. She told the control group nothing. Four weeks later there were no changes to the control group; however, the test group had decreased in weight, blood pressure, body fat, waist-to-hip ratio, and body mass index. Their work hadn't changed, so it seems that some new thinking or belief in the hotel workers had been enough to change their bodies.

What were the stories that these elderly men and hotel housekeepers were telling themselves? How did their body and brain change so much just by their thoughts? Almost everything you've learned about having a baby and maybe breastfeeding was learned "mindlessly" years ago before you had the benefit of insight and positive stories. Now you do and now you can change that old habit of thought by relearning mindfully for a positive birth and parenting experience. Optimists have a can-do positive attitude and pessimists tend to focus on what they can't do. A Mayo Clinic study indicates that optimists on average live longer than pessimists do. Penn State University tracked 120 men who had suffered one heart attack. After eight years, they found that 80% of pessimists had died of a second attack, compared with 33% of optimists. Other research suggests that optimism can lead to success at work school and sports and we know it's an important aspect of preparing for a big event like having a baby and becoming a parent.

THE GENTLEBIRTH MINDSET

One of the biggest determining factors in how you will handle a challenging event is how you think about your ability to cope with the challenges - your mindset. This sentence is worth reading several times...let it sink in. The way you envision yourself in labor will impact how your labor unfolds. Right now when you imagine yourself in labor what does that scene look like? As if you're watching yourself on TV ... are you calm and focused with your confident, well-trained partner by your side? Do you feel strong and determined? If it is then you already have a head start! But it's very possible that what you're actually imagining is you wailing on a bed, feeling out of control and terrified with your partner frozen in fear. The good news is that all is not lost if you're currently 'rehearsing' a less than positive birth experience. It means you're going to get even more out of this book. I'll give you a free pass on this occasion as you're brand new to GentleBirth but shifting your mindset begins today – right now with you noticing what stories are playing out in your mind when you think about your baby's birth...breastfeeding...parenting.

A mindset is a filter or lens that colors every experience you have. It is a set of beliefs that shape your reality including physical reactions. We have a constant running commentary going on in our mind as our brain is always monitoring and interpreting the world around us our experiences but sometimes the interpretation isn't accurate especially when we take things personally. Mindsets frame the running commentary in a negative or positive way. The GentleBirth mindset creates an internal voice focused on positive expectations seeing birth and parenting as a challenge - a challenge we can prepare for and become confident in our abilities.

When we explore the mindset research it's suggested that there are two kinds one that is fixed or growth (flexible mindset). A fixed mindset is a voice that says things like "It's going to be so awful – I just know I won't cope, I shouldn't set my expectations so high...why even try." It's usually quite judgmental too. Parents with a growth mindset are more aware of judging themselves and realize it can be damaging when preparing for our baby's birth. Mindfulness helps parents become aware of that inner voice and which is the dominant mindset – most of us have a mix of both. GentleBirth parents are more focused on taking positive experience and learning from experience to have the most positive birth possible. They adopt a more curious adaptable attitude.

When we look at mindset and stress the ideal stress response gives us energy and focus and motivates us to act in a way that is healthy - it is a motivator to help us reach our goals – a positive birth and parenting experience. You might be familiar with the fight/flight response (panic and fear) and the oxytocin response (calm and connected) but there is another stress response – the challenge-response – aka the 'excite and delight' response. You can learn how to transform a fight/flight response into a challenge-response. Is adrenaline all bad? Only if it's constant and part of fight or flight. The challenge-response is healthier for you and your baby. No study shows that an absence of stress response improves our lives as nice as it sounds. We can't eliminate stress but we can transform it. All studies show the stress response is enhanced with the presence of the challenge-response. So how does that translate into preparing for birth? There is a fine line between feeling excited and running from a scary bear but you can 'get good' at stress.

A University of New Orleans study compared novice and experienced skydivers...you might think that the experienced skydivers would have a lower heart rate given their years of experience but their heart rate was higher. The more excited they were the bigger their 'excite and delight' response. We're approaching birth/parenting as a challenge. We recognize that your true potential is unknown but a positive birth is 100% achievable with the right mindset during one of the most challenging times of your life. In the challenge-response your body acts as if you're exercising...your blood vessels expand and your critical thinking brain remains active. In a fight/flight response, the blood vessels constrict making our body and brain work against us in labor. Emotionally you feel afraid and that primary goal is to protect and survive...in a challenge-response, you feel excited and energized...it's not about escaping a threat but going after what you want – and rocking your birth! A little anxiety is a good thing especially in the last few weeks of pregnancy – you're about to go through a huge life-changing experience. Surgeons are more focused and have improved fine motor skills in a challenge-response. Studies also show that pilots have safer landings in a flight simulator when the challenge-response is initiated as they can access the neo-cortex (the critical thinking part of the brain). Right from the beginning of your pregnancy (or starting today) immerse yourself in positive birth stories and get your birth team in place. Focus on your resources and previous experiences overcoming stressful events. We always see a huge mindset shift after our workshops. You start to engage the challenge-response and are ready to rock your birth. When labor starts that fast beating heart means you are getting ready to take on that challenge – it is oxygenating your muscles and bringing nutrients to your body for the work of labor. Reframing that fast beating heart is essential - it is giving you energy rather than panic. It's so much easier to move from challenge-response to calm and connected – especially in early labor when it's important to conserve energy.

Here are a couple of ways to cultivate your new mindset for stress. This is not just for labor but for life.

Notice the stress – notice how it's affecting you…just noticing it means you can do something about it.

Recognize that stress is letting you know this is something you really care about.

Learn from any setbacks or bumps in the road and control the controllables.

Be aware of your internal voice and act on it based on your individual preferences…maybe that is to change birth preferences, find a new care-provider, hire a doula etc.

Try to tune into the helpful and unhelpful voices in your head and practice focusing and acting on the growth mindset (here's a hint – it's the internal narrator that makes you feel good).

▌WHAT IS YOUR MINDSET TODAY?

Being able to identify our dominant mindset is really helpful. My youngest son Cooper has been learning about mindset in school and it's making a huge difference to his confidence. If you think you have a fixed mindset don't worry you can learn how to channel those thoughts into a more positive mindset. Let me help you do that.

A parent with a more fixed mindset would say something like "I don't think I can do this, I don't think I can even try."

A growth mindset would say. "I don't know if I can do this but I will stack the odds in my favor and learn more so I can build my birth toolkit."

A fixed mindset would have more thoughts like 'what if you scream in labor, what will everyone think – I'll be so embarrassed'.

A growth mindset would say – 'lots of GentleBirth moms make noise in labor – it can be a great coping mechanism – think of the tennis players and weight lifters who use sounds to help them.'

A fixed mindset would say – 'if you don't try you can just keep your dignity... and no embarrassment...what will your family think'?

A growth mindset would be thinking – 'If I don't give it my best shot I'll never know what my limits are or how strong I am - does it matter what my family thinks? I will know that I will have done my best for my baby'.

A fixed mindset would say – 'I should just do what the doctor says'...a growth mindset would say ' I am the expert on my baby – basketball wasn't easy for Michael Jordan but he was committed and what the nurse suggested just didn't feel right for me – I think I need to ask for more information.'

When feeling criticized a fixed mindset would say 'it wasn't my fault'....it was someone else's or something else's fault. A mom with a growth mindset would say 'if I don't take responsibility I can't make improvements – they mean well and I'll listen to them – I'm sure I can take away something positive'.

As you become aware of these voices you'll see where your focus is... and adjust it in the coming weeks. When you can hear both voices and then act on the growth mindset your whole experience of pregnancy and parenting will change. See how it works for you over the coming weeks. Listen in to your own self-talk and determine what your mindset is and whether you lean toward a growth or fixed mindset....and as you listen in ...challenge some of

those fixed thoughts and consider what action can you take to move toward a more growth-focused mindset.

Use the 3 Ps Throughout Your Pregnancy

- **Focus on the Present**
- **Focus on the Positive**
- **Focus on the Process**

THE CHAMPIONS MINDSET FOR MOTHERHOOD

Muhammad Ali was only 22 years of age when he fought Sonny Liston. Back then – boxing experts relied on physical measurements called tales of the tape to determine how good a boxer was. It measured reach, weight, chest measurements, fist size. However, Ali didn't really measure up – at least physically. Experts didn't give him a chance. Sonny Liston seemed to have it all ...the matchup was so ludicrous the arena was only half full. Apart from Ali's speed, his mind was his biggest asset. He studied Sonny and tried to get into Sonny Liston's mind and then turned it against him. Why did Ali appear to go crazy before each fight? The most powerful punch was the one you didn't see coming. Ali wanted Liston to think he was mentally unstable and was capable of anything so he played on Sonny's fears. According to Ali speaking about Liston, 'all he could see was all mouth...that was all I wanted him to see'. Ali definitely looked powerful but his mind was even more powerful. When you look at photos of Ali we tend to think about his physical fitness instead of his mental fitness. His heart rate and blood pressure were off the chart right before the fight and it was almost canceled... (sounds like a challenge-response to me - this was not fight flight or panic...this was Ali getting ready to rock Sonny Liston's world). He predicted he would win in 8 but he won in 6. He used little rhymes to upset his competitors....'round 8 to prove I'm great'.

Another elite athlete, Michael Jordan the NBA basketball player had a unique mindset. He never made the school team or the first NBA teams. According to Jordan, "the mental toughness and heart are a lot stronger than the physical advantage you might have." But most people only see the physical perfection that led to his greatness, not his mindset. The GentleBirth mindset continues to astound me - the confidence that GentleBirth parents exude after a workshop especially when they are faced with setbacks...there is no question that these moms have had a shift in mindset and the partners too. They leave the workshop filled with confidence that they will be able to handle the challenges ahead – there is an unwavering belief that they can handle anything that comes their way on the big day.

HOW TO STOP NEGATIVE THINKING IN PREGNANCY

You can't. The end.

Trying to NOT think about that time you embarrassed yourself in front of the whole office just doesn't work. And trying to suppress thoughts about pooping in labor is like holding a beach ball under water...it will come back to hit you in the face (the beach ball not the poop). Suppressed thoughts rebound even more intensively and more frequently. In this segment, you're going to learn lots of simple strategies that with a little practice can raise your level of pregnancy and parenting enjoyment significantly. Leaning on your partner during pregnancy and the postpartum weeks is important but wouldn't it be wonderful to have even more of your own inner resources available to you in those few months.

Ok so you can't just stop every single negative thought you have but you can avoid hanging with the Negative Nellies.

Imagine you have a few weeks to your EDD (aka your guess date) and you are so excited for labor to begin you can't stand it. Then one day during lunch a colleague starts throwing shade about how she took one of those 'natural birth' classes and it all went out the window as soon as she felt that first contraction and reminds you that there's 'no medals for going without'…. (you get the picture).

Conversations with NNs (Negative Nellies) are exhausting. Before you know it you've taken the bait. You find yourself defending your choices, digging your heels in and ultimately putting more pressure on yourself as you resolve to "show them".

It takes self restraint but the more you engage with these Negative Nellies you'll find yourself being less blissed and more stressed in the coming weeks.

STRATEGIES FOR DEALING WITH NEGATIVE NELLIES

Avoid them whenever possible. Research shows that repeated exposure to stimuli that causes strong negative emotions is bad for your health (and your baby's). Think of it this way - if the Negative Nelly was a smoker would you sit there through your lunch break and inhale their second-hand smoke? Nope.

If you can't avoid them and have to work with them at a minimum avoid discussions about birth/breastfeeding and vaccinations. These are a sure fire way to poke the mama bear. When they ask if you're getting the epidural just smile and say "I'm not ruling it out. We'll see how we go on the day". Then quickly change the topic to Game of Thrones.

Find your positive birth 'tribe' – it takes a village but it's the village idiots that you need to watch out for. Hang out with likeminded moms in person and virtually.

If you've been to a GentleBirth class your partner will know the importance of running interference on these kinds of discussions at family gatherings. These are a hot spot for NNs so be alert especially if you're a first time mom. NNs have a built in tracking system to find you and make you miserable. Most of the time your Cocoon of Calm practice can render you invisible to their radar – the more practice you do the less penetrable your cocoon is to them (like water off a ducks back).

Choose your battles: Your OB suggests that giving birth on the bed is easier for everyone and he can prevent you having a tear. Smile and nod....and smile even more as you change to a more supportive hospital/OB/Midwife.

Don't take it personally NNs haven't had the benefit of brain training for birth to rewire their brains so they're not as emotionally and mentally fit for birth as you are. When the Negative Nellies throw down the gauntlet – take a breath and step over it (this is a great opportunity to practice slow controlled breathing).

Be kind, it's not your job to turn everyone into Positive Pollies – that's mine.

Share the love and recommend my book to them.

▌MEDITATION – IT'S NOT WHAT YOU THINK

In the next few pages I'm going to share some of the benefits of meditation (and there are plenty) but if you have an aversion to what you *think* meditation is and are about to skip ahead to signs of labor here it is.

> *In a nutshell*
>
> *Yes there are plenty of demonstrated benefits from learning how to meditate but they are secondary to the real reason meditation is such an important tool for women in particular. Practicing meditation helps you notice all the BS the voice in your head tries to convince you is true. This is as far from a relaxation technique as you can get. If you can get to grips in pregnancy with the fact that your mind lies to you – you have NO IDEA how much more empowered you'll feel in those long challenging weeks after your baby arrives. When that voice is telling you what a crap mom you are, how awful your body looks (insert additional various insults here) and you realize you don't have to take the bait - it's life changing.*

The Scene: Tracy the Midwife is frantically trying to finish up a project that was due yesterday. She hasn't eaten since early morning – it's now 2.40pm

Actors: Tracy (played by herself)

VIMH (Voice in My Head) played by my judgy mind.

Tracy: Sh*t I forgot to pick up Jack from school (as she frantically grabs her keys and races to the car).

VIMH: Ugh AGAIN??? You're such a crap mom, how can any mother forget to pick up their own kid from school? You suck.

Tracy: I must be the only mom to ever do this. I suck (metaphorically beats herself with a big stick for perceived parenting inadequacies).

VIMH: Can't argue there, no awards for mother of the year for you. What if he's kidnapped – how could you live with yourself if something happened to him?

These kinds of 'conversations' are happening every waking hour, so although the scene may be different for you the tone is usually arsey (unkind, mean, critical and judgy). When you practice meditation the scene and how you feel about the scene changes.

VIMH (Voice in My Head) played by my judgy mind.

Tracy: Sh*t I forgot to pick Jack up from school (as she frantically grabs her keys and races to the car).

VIMH: Ugh AGAIN? You're such a crap mom, how can any mother forget to pick up their own kid from school? You suck.

Tracy: Well hello to you too evil twin, it's been a while. I was wondering when you'd show up again. Thank you for 'insightful' feedback on my parenting skills as always but I think I'll cut myself some slack today. It's been a crazy day and Jack is 14 not 4 – waiting an extra 10 minutes at school isn't the end of the world. Sh*t happens and I'm not the first mom to ever do this and I definitely won't be the last.

VIMH: Errrr ok (hair flip and VIHM exits stage left).

Scene fades – Tracy notices the unwanted negative opinion of her 'evil twin' (more on that later) and with a friendly but no nonsense attitude cuts the interaction short and cuts herself some slack.

Meditation makes your mind a stage – and your thoughts and feelings are the actors but you get to see who the actors are (the evil ones tend to read from the same judgy script). Just like great Pantomimes the character we love (awareness) will help you see the villains 'it's BEHIND YOU' when VIMH tries to sneak up on you and hijack your wellbeing.

Are you still with me? Good then let's learn more.

NO MOUNTAIN TOP REQUIRED

You probably think your mind is too busy to practice meditation or you're too strong willed, too fidgety or you think you have to listen to pan pipes. The word "mindfulness" can bring up images of sitting cross-legged in front of crystals chanting 'OM' while silently wrestling with your mind to stop thinking. It's not a religion and it requires no special clothing or difficult training. But it does take patience, persistence and a very forgiving attitude. As someone who multitasks in my sleep, calming my brain 'chatter' can be hard work. Sitting still for five minutes without your phone, TV, or iPad can be challenging for many of us these days. Remember that last time your Wi-Fi went down during an important project (or TV show)... amplify that feeling x 10. Not a good feeling.

Most of us tend to go through life on autopilot with our head in the past, reliving a past experience, or in the future, worrying about what's going to happen. We have to learn how to train ourselves to let stressful thoughts go and stop trying to wrestle with our minds to change the way we think we 'should' feel about pregnancy, birth, and parenting especially if you're not enjoying this time in your life as much as you think you should. Mindfulness in a nutshell is about focus – where you put it determines how good you feel and I'll take a wild guess that feeling good is important to you.

"Let thoughts come and go.
Just don't serve them tea."
–Shunryn Suzuki–

In other words don't spend too much time entertaining these unwelcome 'visitors' especially if they are stressing you out. Before I started meditating I used to not just serve them tea but a whole four-course meal, I still do it every so often – some days are just easier than others.

In every single experience you have in pregnancy and, as a new parent, there are three basic elements; Your thoughts, your feelings and the sensations in your body. As you're reading this page you're having thoughts about what you're reading or maybe you're thinking about dinner. You may also be having an emotional response to a birth story and you're also experiencing some sensations in your body (you just might not have been aware of them until I mentioned it). Maybe you're feeling your baby's kicks...or your back feels stiff. When you are feeling anxious you can probably feel your heart beating faster and your breathing getting faster. When you are meditating we start with these three elements. Remember - thoughts, feelings and sensations are the key to mindfulness practice.

In a fascinating experiment, a group of participants was given the choice between sitting in a room alone with their thoughts for several minutes with no distractions or they could choose to give themselves a mild electric shock – ¼ of the women and 2/3 of the men chose to zap themselves. (Answers the question of which sex is the more 'evolved'). The researchers did find some correlation between mindfulness and the ability to entertain ourselves. I'll take a short mindfulness session over an electric shock any day (wonder what my husband thinks...).

AUTOPILOT

Your brain has a brilliant way of creating 'shortcuts' that makes your life so much easier. Imagine having to learn how to walk every morning, or how to drive your car? Thankfully once you've mastered these skills your brain creates a shortcut (like a shortcut you might have on your desktop) to access certain programs. These shortcuts free up our brain's resources so you can multitask, but we're now learning that all of this multitasking that we've become so used to bragging about may not be all that healthy for us.

See how often you can catch yourself on autopilot today. We've all had the experiences of putting our keys down and not being able to find them or walking into a room and forgetting what you went in there for. It would be easy to blame this on pregnancy brain but this is also you running on autopilot – you are so immersed in the next activity or what happened yesterday that you are physically doing the actions but you're not "there." Mindfulness just means you are being present on purpose you're paying attention to what you're doing at this very moment - on purpose. You are choosing to be completely absorbed in your current activity brushing your teeth having a shower washing the dishes. These may not be the most exciting activities of your life but paying attention to them as you do them stops your mind jumping from the past into the future looking for all the regrettable decisions you've ever made.

For just a moment or two, notice where your feet are. Are they connected to the floor? Can you feel the carpet under your feet? Or maybe you can notice the temperature of your toes. Now notice the way your back feels against the chair, don't change position, just notice it. See - you're practicing mindfulness already and not a whiff of incense in the air! Take baby steps and try being mindful while you're drinking your coffee today; notice the temperature on your lips and tongue, the taste or, as you walk to your car, notice how your muscles move effortlessly over the ground. Sense how your feet feel in your shoes ... are they warm or cold? As you take a bite of your sandwich - slow down and really taste the different flavors the textures how your jaw chews and the sensation of swallowing that bite. Savor the taste and, more important, savor the moment. Mindlessness (autopilot) is a habit, an unhealthy one, but mindfulness is like a muscle that gets stronger the more you practice. Try a few of these exercises today and notice how your mind itches to run away as soon as you take your focus away from that moment. When you notice your mind making a quick exit to think of all the things it believes you should be doing, be easy with yourself - just gently move your awareness back to that delicious sandwich.

So, as you have no doubt experienced, even in the previous simple exercises, your mind loves to wander. It loves to spend time in the past replaying events that have already happened thinking about what we should have said how things could have been different etc., etc. It also loves worrying about things that will most likely never happen. In GentleBirth we say, "Do not feed the fears." Most of what we worry about never happens.

Mindfulness isn't just a nice "to do" for yourself that makes you feel relaxed. With practice, the physical structure of your brain can change in as little as 8 weeks. Being mindful doesn't mean stopping your thoughts. It's about noticing them, noticing how you react to them, and then, in some cases, changing that reaction. Mindfulness teachers often talk about the practice of mindfulness helping you become more 'awake' in your life (being present and not on autopilot) – trust me you're about to be very 'awake' in your life in the coming months...3am...4am...5am – using these tools won't make your baby sleep but they'll help you adapt to the intensity of emotions that come with these changes.

MEDITATION AND MINDFULNESS

Think of meditation as an umbrella term for different types of mindfulness – just like 'sports' includes running, gymnastics and swimming. Meditation is considered the 'on cushion' time (couch, chair, bed...all are fine too) when you take the time out of your day to literally sit and practice. Mindfulness is an approach to life where you are learning how to pay more attention to what's happening right now throughout the day instead of letting autopilot and the negativity bias run the show. There are multiple benefits physically and psychologically for the practice of both and if you're using the GentleBirth App you'll see I take a very gentle approach to the sitting meditation as it's such a new concept in today's multitasking, instant gratification culture. If you have 5 minutes to spend watching cute baby goats in pajamas on YouTube you have time to practice 5 minutes of mindfulness today. Seriously – just 5 minutes, and to begin with we're going to set the bar really low so you can't fail and if 5 minutes is a stretch try 1 minute instead. Let's keep our expectations low too while you get settled into a few minutes practice each day.

Just start with noticing your breath – as you breathe in where do you feel it? How about as you breathe out? Where do you notice the exhalation? A few seconds into the meditation your brain is going to be hijacked by a thought and then another and another and it usually goes something like this.

Tracy: This is boring...kinda hungry...I'm always hungry these days, have to start eating healthier, why did I eat that second brownie I'll never lose the pregnancy weight.

Tracy: Hmm chocolate brownies...or a nice salted caramel brownie... with a cool glass of milk...man I'm thirsty.

Tracy: I think I read somewhere that always feeling thirsty is a sign of diabetes? Maybe I have Gestational Diabetes...

Tracy: OMG if I have Gestational Diabetes I might need a cesarean.

Tracy: Sh*t I'm supposed to be noticing my breath. Better start again.

Tracy: I'm pathetic ...it was only one minute and I failed already. I'll have a piece of chocolate after I finish as my reward. I heard chocolate is a good source of iron and if I'm having a cesarean I'll need healthy iron levels.

A MINDFUL FRAMEWORK FOR PREGNANCY AND BEYOND

Meditation is so much more than just breathing. There are specific 'pillars' or attitudes that can reduce the stress in your life considerably. They are all interconnected, so it's not a checklist of mindful tasks but another layer of richness that you can allow to be part of your pregnancy as you begin to pay more attention to your thoughts and feelings in pregnancy. Depending on what you've got going on in your pregnancy now you might find that you're drawn to one of these 'attitudes' and next week a different aspect may resonate more with you.

Beginner's Mind: This is what happens when you intentionally try to look at things with fresh eyes and without the 'story'. The 'story' is whatever running commentary is running through your mind all day every day. When we're on autopilot we miss the richness of our experience. Beginner's mind means to notice the world around us with curiosity and openness, as if you've just arrived from Mars and this is the first time you see, hear, feel, taste, or experience this or your brand new baby experiencing life on the outside for the very first time. In new experiences, it's easier to have a beginner's mind like when you go to a new restaurant and you take in all of the details and you really taste your food. When was the last time you adopted the same curious attitude to your Saturday night take-out or your commute to work? You'll be surprised at how much you're missing when you're lost in thought mentally battling your mother in law.

NON-JUDGMENT - DON'T BECOME THE JUDGY MOM

You see a mom in the supermarket loading up her shopping cart with junk food and trying to wrangle her toddler who is having the mother of all meltdowns. Within seconds you've mentally clocked that she can't control her kids or her eating habits all without so much as a hello. Sound familiar? Let's get real - you already are a judgy mom, no matter how much you like to think otherwise. We all judge, that's what the brain does. It is normal neurological functioning of that amazing organ in your skull handed down from our ancestors when it could mean life or death to make a split second judgment on who might be friend or foe. So when someone tries to tell you how non-judgmental they are it's like saying I'm a 'non-thinker or a non-breather'. If you are alive and have normal brain functioning you're judgy. In a split second, we also automatically compare everything in our experience throughout the day. I bet if you've ever tried to meditate in the past the judgments were quick and harsh and might have even left you feeling like you're the worst meditator in the world. We're mentally liking or disliking everything around us from the moment you first open your eyes. We judge everything as good or bad, wanted or unwanted, beautiful or ugly. As humans we prefer to have all the nice things in our lives, we want the sunny weather, we want our boss to be in a good mood, we love it when the train is on time. But when that winter storm comes through and you have to scrape the ice off the windscreen or when your manager's mood sends you cubicle jumping to avoid bumping into them or when that train is late AGAIN all bets are off. In an instant, we believe the world has turned against us and is punishing us for less than wholesome deeds from a past life.

▌DON'T SHOOT THE SECOND ARROW

When things aren't going our way it's not just the icy windscreen or late train that stresses us out – it's the story we tell ourselves about that event that adds an extra layer of insult to injury. It's known as the 'second arrow'. In the Buddhist teachings it's said that any time we experience something negative, two arrows fly towards us. The first arrow is the actual event itself (the late train), which is annoying in itself. The second arrow is how you respond to the first arrow i.e. keeping that annoying feeling going and building on it until you're in a rage when the train arrives and fume all the way home. But you see the second arrow is always optional. You can choose to respond differently.

Maybe that stream of thought goes something like this "I can't believe this... I'm going to be late and the whole team is going to be annoyed. I should have checked the weather last night and gotten up a bit earlier to defrost the windscreen. Why did Paul insist on getting this car? I should have paid extra and gotten the one with the instant clear. He should have researched this better, he doesn't research anything properly. I can't even get him to come with me to buy the stroller. Maria's husband is so thoughtful and wants to be so involved in all of the preparations. What kind of dad is Paul going to be?" So you can see how one frosty windscreen has gone from a minor inconvenience to re-evaluating your partner's commitment to you in about 60 seconds and quite possibly a frosty encounter with your partner tonight.

What can you do?

The last thing I want you to do is to start judging your judging. You'll never stop your brain from comparing, so let's work with it instead. Notice your judging in an easy-going way; I say something like 'Hmmm, you have your judgy hat on right now, Tracy,' so I'm able to catch myself (most of the time) before I add on the unnecessary stress of the story my mind is about to launch into about how the world has done me wrong. Then I bring my attention back to whatever I was doing at the time. Have a friendly, curious attitude to all of these concepts and they will serve you well. Think of everything in this book as an interesting experiment.

▌ACCEPTANCE

"Pregnancy is a process that invites you to surrender to the unseen force behind all life."
–Judy Ford–

Another game-changer – if you want to really enjoy the next few months and stress a whole lot less when your baby is here this is a must do. These four words;

THIS TOO SHALL PASS – memorize them...tattoo them to your hand if you need to. At 4am after months of not sleeping you may start to have visions of your college age daughter impersonating a starfish in your bed as you cling to the edge (of the bed and your sanity).

Say it with me – THIS TOO SHALL PASS (works for hemorrhoids, cankles and breastfeeding challenges too).

It will be a skill you will hone as a new parent, so get a head start today. This is an area that most parents say saved their sanity the most in early parenting. The attitude of acceptance can truly be a game-changer in those early weeks of little sleep and diving hormones. Mindful acceptance doesn't mean you become a doormat and roll over when someone is rude to you or suffering physically and mentally by not sleeping for the first 3 years of your child's life. Sometimes there's confusion that acceptance is associated with resignation. Noah Rasheta explains it well; "Acceptance is like sitting in a field, looking up at the sky and watching the clouds go by. There is no resistance to the moment to moment experience, there is only observation and acceptance. It would be silly to watch the clouds and be upset that they are not forming into the specific shapes we want. And yet, that's exactly what we do in life. I like to compare the experience of being alive to the experience of playing a game of Tetris. If you've played Tetris, you know that the whole point of the game is to wait and see what shape will appear next, and then you have to work with it to position it in the best way possible...in order to continue playing the game...isn't that the very game of life? Imagine for a minute that you're watching someone play Tetris...and every time a new shape appears, they go into a tantrum and yell and scream at the game and say "THAT IS NOT THE SHAPE I WAS EXPECTING"..." "THAT IS NOT THE SHAPE I WANTED". HOW SILLY WOULD THAT BE? But isn't that exactly how we tend to play the game of life? Acceptance is like playing a game and not resisting the challenges of that game. Life is the same... Acceptance is being open to the actual feelings we're having in the moment to moment experience of life and being willing to just feel that. Whatever it is...anger, happiness, fear, jealousy, anxiety...We can learn to simply BE with our experience or we can try to control the experience... controlling it is the opposite of acceptance. Anytime we're trying to manipulate our inner experience, we're doing the opposite of accepting it. Think about someone playing Candy Crush and yelling at the game... you'll see how reactivity restricts our ability to accept. Reactivity prevents us from being able to respond. Acceptance is a form of responding instead of reacting. Resignation would be an example of reacting while acceptance would be an example of how we chose to respond. To build your capacity for acceptance, imagine you are a non-judgmental observer or a witness to your thoughts or emotions.

As I mentioned accepting reality can feel like surrendering, but mindful acceptance is not passive, it's active. Acceptance is an intentional willingness to acknowledge reality as it is, which moves us from experiencing emotional distress to choosing a different intentional action. It's not "I can't believe this traffic is so slow! If it doesn't speed up soon I'm going to be late! This is awful and so unfair!" (judgment and resisting reality) or even "This traffic is very slow. I can't change the traffic, nothing can be done. I guess I'll just get there late" (passive surrender), but instead, "This traffic is very slow. I may be late. Hmmm, I could take a different route, or call to let them know. Maybe I will leave earlier next time." Acceptance of what is doesn't mean we always have to like what's happening – we all have limits but when we can allow a situation with more compassion and less judgment it might not change the situation but it'll definitely make it easier to tolerate. Remember this section when it's 4 am and you're three days postpartum and your inner narrator is giving you a million reasons why you shouldn't breastfeed or when your baby is six months old and not sleeping through the night.

Let it Go: As I'm writing this I can hear the theme to *Frozen* (and I bet you can, too – sorry about that). This attitude ties in with so many others and is well worth the practice during your pregnancy. Let go of the 'shoulds' and any unrealistic expectations you have of yourself and of other people. There's a famous saying "replace expectation with appreciation" and you can't go wrong. If you don't get the dishwasher unloaded today can you let that sh*t go and not torture yourself? If you didn't hear your baby crying while you were in the shower for a whole 3 minutes can you not award yourself worst mother in the world title? I can't say this enough if you can adopt a more chillaxed approach to your journey through parenthood you'll save yourself (and your family) a lot of unnecessary tears and torture.

"Take control of your mind and meditate.
Let your soul gravitate to the love, ya'll"
–Black Eyed Peas–

Non-Striving:

You're probably reading this book because you're Type A and goal oriented. Having goals isn't a bad thing but, when we obsessively chase goals that are elusive, we can run into big problems. You're very used to doing instead of being and you judge your achievements or non-achievements with a very critical eye (I have that T-shirt too). You might even find some of the meditation sessions in the App make you a bit twitchy as your mind keeps reminding you of the 2 million other things you could be doing during that 10 minutes of practice. No doubt one of your goals is to be the perfect mom, to have a positive birth experience on the big day and you have certain ideas of how you want that day to go. Then add your internal pressure of what you 'should do' now add the competitive pressures of modern day living – your home 'should' be tidy, you 'should' be able to work full time and raise the perfect family while keeping up your Insta posts of your picture perfect life. The mind is always traveling... reaching or striving to change the present moment instead of paying attention to what's happening at this moment and dropping the shoulds. The 'shoulds' are enemy #1 of motherhood and as you'll see 'shoulding' and 'judging' tend to hang out together quite a bit. So try a little less to be the perfect mom and be more present today – a good enough mom is good enough.

Patience: An understanding and acceptance that sometimes things must unfold in their own time and trying to make it change only makes you more stressed. We live in an instant gratification society and we expect quick solutions to everything. Parenting requires unlimited patience – with yourself and your partner as you adjust to these intense changes. Everyone wants their baby to sleep through the night....but it has to happen at your baby's pace – not the baby book's pace. Many women want to get back to 'normal' after having a baby but this is a new normal and although things may seem intense now they are changing every day.

Give yourself the time to practice, and give yourself the grace to be aware of every emotion you experience as a new parent, whether they are feelings of joy and gratitude or feelings of impatience and frustration.

Trust: Trusting in your intuition (gut feeling).

You'll hear lots of people telling you to trust your gut when it comes to pregnancy and parenting. It sounds very wise but the problem is most of us haven't had a conversation with our gut in a very long time so how can we trust it especially when those voices in our head are running the show and jumping to all the wrong conclusions. We need to be able to tell the difference between our intuition and a fear response (a fear response makes it very difficult to make any kind of rational decision). Because we're so in our heads all of the time it can be difficult to hear any of the other sources of knowledge that our body is trying to share with us but as you practice more and more getting out of your head and into your body you'll have more opportunities to connect with a quieter place where you can learn to hear what your instincts are telling you.

Gratitude

It's just good manners to say thank you and you'll spend a lot of time trying to get your toddler to say it. When you take a minute to check in with all the good stuff going on in your life it makes stress take a back seat.

I know for me when it's 7:30am on a Monday morning and I'm getting the boys in the car to get to school being grateful is so easy when the sun is shining and the traffic is light...but it's a bit harder when you're late, it's pouring rain and the traffic is at a standstill. You can't feel appreciation and stress at the same time. Don't believe me? Just try it. An attitude of gratitude is like an off switch for whatever greatest hits of stressful thoughts you're currently playing.

BIRTH STORY

This day 6 years ago, my 2nd GentleBirth baby was born. I remember it like it was yesterday. I had a late appointment with the midwives clinic in Holles St and had a feeling I was going to be having a baby that night. I must have been convincing because the midwife said, go up and get checked, mum is usually right. My first labor was only 6 hours long and we lived an hour from the hospital at the time, so she said she'd like me to get checked rather than go home as chances are it'd be quicker this time. I went up, they checked me and said my cervix was high and unfavorable and that I'd most likely be back in for an appointment the following week.

Off I went home to put my 20 month old to bed and to get myself organized for hospital as I just KNEW something was going on. I had a bath in clary sage oil, felt uncomfortable so got out and had a shower and put my PJs on. I told himself to make sure to have his bag packed and to go to the shop for sweets as he was caught short last time. I was blow drying my hair when suddenly my waters went and I was like, well I guess I should go in now. I went downstairs to tell my parents what was going on and they waved me off and I was putting one leg into the car to sit down when suddenly a MASSIVE burst of waters came out and I could feel the urge to push. GAAAAH! There were noises coming from me that I never knew I could make and I went back inside and went on all fours. Hubby had called an ambulance.

I was so quiet then, just willing the baby not to come as I chased everyone out of the room and cursed myself for not vacuuming the floor, thinking he was going to be born onto crumbs and fluff. I remember clearly watching the weather forecast after the 9 o'clock news. The ambulance came within minutes and they looked briefly down my PJs and said "nah you're grand but come on in, we'll bring you". They made me lie down on the stretcher inside the ambulance and I just breathed and breathed. I could see my belly going nuts but wasn't really in pain - my TENS was on by this point. We made it to O'Connell Bridge and they stopped and told me they could see the head crowning so I could push and I said no, sure the hospital is just over there, let's just go. Off we went again and they were waiting for me there, key to the lift in hand and I was brought up to delivery room. They lifted me from the stretcher to the bed and the midwife said, ok, let's see how far along you are and she looked and laughed and said ok, you can push. So I finally felt OK to push and in one push he slid out, 8lbs exactly. My boy. He was born at 5mins to 10. I'd been on the floor watching the weather forecast at 9.30! My gorgeous George.

I panicked when I felt the urge to push in the driveway just after my waters broke the second time, but after that I totally went into a zone where I was absolutely working with him to stay safe and calm. We were the perfect team and I can honestly say it was one of the best experiences of my life, along with my first and my third delivery. So thank you Tracy for giving me such an amazing gift, one I can cherish for as long as I live. GentleBirth has given me so much and I'm so envious of anyone who has yet to go through labor as my baby is now 4 and our family is complete.

Aine

HOW MORGAN FREEMAN MADE ME A BETTER MOM

We all have that internal 'narrator' in our heads (some people call it their evil twin). It's like an ongoing newscast that's usually kinda critical and judges everything you do every minute of your waking day. Part of it is just how our brains work but a larger part of this ongoing unhelpful commentary is a habit of thought. We tend to hear this mean newscaster loudest when we hit our teens and, after a while, we don't notice it as much but if you pay attention you can start to hear it again. These narrators show up in pregnancy quite vocally too and if you don't fire them they'll hang around to derail your intentions for being the best mom you can be.

For most of us, our narrators sound like Alan Rickman or some other villainous, catty character. I had a chorus of Alan Rickman (Severus Snape) Jack Nicholson ("you can't handle the truth"), and other less than gentle commentators after I had Jack. I never realized that Morgan Freeman was sitting in the wings just waiting for an invitation to step forward onto the stage of my mind and change my entire outlook on breastfeeding, mothering and the world in general. I had to learn not to fight that annoying narrator but just to notice my evil twin's commentary and say to myself "there she goes again (evil twin again) – she's on a roll today".

One of the biggest challenges for a new breastfeeding mom is the way you think about breastfeeding (those commentators have strong opinions about how things SHOULD be done). The way you think about breastfeeding has been heavily influenced by how others think about it... those who have breastfed and those who haven't. Thinking in itself isn't the problem. Believing everything you think IS! We get so caught up in the thoughts and expectations about being a mom, but you are not your thoughts or feelings... you can learn how to step back and, like a camera lens, pan out to see what's really going on, watch the thoughts and choose a different response. You also get to choose a more gentle, compassionate narrator to help you along the way.

Before you became a mom your expectations about breastfeeding probably went something like this "your partner arrives in from work as you're snuggling by the fire with your calm and quiet newborn as she drinks in that liquid gold....her body gets heavier in your arms as she drifts off into peaceful slumber full and content.......you place her gently into her bassinet and you settle in for some quiet time with your partner and catch up on the day, satisfied after a fulfilling nourishing day of blissful mothering". Lovely thoughts indeed but not reality for most of us. More like your partner arrives in from work to an exhausted, teary mom and crying baby...angry exchanges begin starting with "you're late!" Your bewildered partner asks – "Is there any dinner?" ...we all know how that story ends.

For many, this is the reality of those intense few weeks adjusting to your new arrival. The reality is that for most moms it is HARD. So those ideas of what breastfeeding SHOULD be like need to be retired (your evil twin loves 'shoulding' it in your face). Arguing with reality won't change it and thinking it 'should' be a different way will only make you more unhappy.... you'll waste so much time and energy continuing to struggle with reality ... desperately trying to wrestle 'reality' to the ground and make it into something else but that's not happening.

This is the third night in a row you've been up with an unsettled baby and you are exhausted. Your train of thought is probably something like "not AGAIN......what am I doing wrong? I'm so tired. Is it my milk? Maybe she's not getting enough? What if she's starving? Why is this so hard? Everyone else's babies seem to be sleeping. Why can't she just sleep?? I'm just not able to do this. I'm getting the bottles tomorrow and Paul can get up and feed him. I don't get a break all day and he gets to sleep. I just want her to sleep. I hate my life." And this all happens in the space of about 2 seconds. You'll notice that your evil twin is quite judgmental...critical and not very gentle. Notice how your train of negative thoughts is now picking up speed...(thanks to those nasty narrators). When we fall into the habit of responding to a stressful situation on autopilot it's like you've fallen asleep on the train (of thought). You wake up and realize you've gone way past your stop and it's taking you miles and miles away from where you should be. You get to decide if you'll stay on the train taking you further away from your intended destination (to be the best mom you can be) or get off at the next stop and head back so you can take some mindful action if necessary to help solve your sleep/ breastfeeding challenges.

Along with the self-critical judgmental thoughts, you're also probably experiencing the unsettling emotions of frustration, anger, sadness maybe even inadequacy. You feel short-changed...hard done by. This is NOT what you thought you were signing up for!

Physically your heart rate is increasing, you may have a knot in your stomach...your breathing has quickened. Your body is tightly wound.

Your thoughts about what's happening have become a runaway train picking up speed and heading for disaster, they've triggered a cascade of emotional responses and kicked off the stress response. You feel overwhelmed, mentally, emotionally and physically and there's just no room to think rationally and take mindful action and you're far from connected to your baby on this runaway train.

Mindfulness can't help you change the situation but it can help you become more gentle (with yourself and your baby) when things are happening that are out of your control. You can meet the challenges without immediately reacting to them. With practice, it gives you a stable base to act from so you can be the mom you intended to be. It doesn't make the thoughts/feelings go away, but it changes how you relate to those thoughts and feelings...nothing is good or bad... it just is. Mindfulness is usually defined as a moment-to-moment non-judgmental awareness of the present moment and meeting it with gentleness and compassion and meeting things the way they are. It doesn't mean you have to like what's happening (especially at 3 am).

When you become a mother so much unnecessary pain is caused by the idea that things 'should' be a certain way (according to the experts...the books....your past experiences and expectations). The idea that things aren't as they 'should' is a pathway to ongoing unnecessary pain and suffering. "It 'should' be different and until it's different I can't be happy". Breastfeeding 'should' be easier than this...millions of women breastfeed every day I 'should' be able to do this. The reality is that right now it's not easy for you, you're having problems getting baby to latch etc...and you need to decide what to do next. How can you meet this experience as it is and find a solution from a calmer, gentler place? That's where Morgan Freeman can help.

In similar circumstances when you feel upset in some way notice that train of thought...the 'shoulds'...and the ever-present judging self-critical mind...take a few breaths...pay attention to how those thoughts show up in your body...and let's go through an experience together approaching it like you would your best friend.

MINDFULNESS OF THOUGHTS, EMOTIONS, AND SENSATIONS

What's Happening Right Now: The baby won't sleep and now he's not latching.

Thoughts & Emotions: "I'm so exhausted. I'm angry with my son and I feel guilty for being annoyed with him – he's only a baby. This shouldn't be so hard...breastfeeding is 'supposed' to be natural. I'm angry that I'm finding this so hard. Nobody tells you how hard it is. It's so frustrating that he just won't do what he's 'supposed' to do. I really wanted to breastfeed but I can't keep going like this. I'm getting bottles tomorrow and Paul can do some feeds so I can sleep. I can't believe I'm such a failure at breastfeeding, how come my sister found it so easy?"

Body: My body is tense, my face feels red, and my breathing is really fast.

What's the real problem with this scenario?

You are tired.

Your baby is hungry.

It's the middle of the night and she won't latch properly.

This is all that's happening right now.

Are you liking what's happening? Nope!

But the latch can nearly always be fixed...babies do eventually sleep more. These are temporary problems. The problem isn't that you're tired (yes, it definitely sucks and nobody enjoys being exhausted.) or that your baby isn't latching properly. The problem is the way you're thinking about it. It's a train of thought but you get to decide if you'll stay on that train.

If you were talking to your best friend in this situation what would you say to her? Maybe something like this (in your best Morgan Freeman voice):

"Take a deep breath. You're ok. It can be really stressful when they won't latch on right away. This is a really intense time in your life and you're exhausted. This is how your daughter communicates with you. It can be so hard in the beginning but you're doing great. Why don't you call a breastfeeding counselor in the morning and get some help?" Talking to yourself gently and mindfully like your best friend would talk to you (or Morgan Freeman) takes practice. You have to catch yourself being critical...often we don't even notice we're doing it because this running commentary has been going on for so long, but if you pay attention you'll feel it in your gut.

In pregnancy and parenting, so many things feel out of control. Your body is doing strange things. Your hormones are making you weepy. Your baby is doing what newborns do (not sleeping). Pregnancy is a great time to start practicing mindfulness so you get the hang of this skill long before your baby arrives. You're learning that, instead of trying to control the uncontrollable (wrestling with reality), it's so much easier to learn how to think about these uncontrollables differently. You can't always change your outer world but you can always change your inner world.

Your MF – Mindfulness (Morgan Freeman) practice can help you increase your tolerance for stressful moments with your baby, partner and the world in general and approach mothering from a more compassionate, gentle place.

The next time you find the Negative Nellies (Alan Rickman et al) going for the jugular:

- Take a few deep breaths...just focus on your breathing especially the pause between breaths.
- Notice what thoughts you're having i.e. "I don't have enough milk."
- Notice the feelings you're experiencing: Frustration, sadness, anger, irritation, fear, and guilt.
- Notice the body sensations that accompany these thoughts/feelings: tightness, knots, racing heart.

When you focus on your breathing for a few moments that train of thought keeps going but it doesn't pick up speed, it loses momentum. You can watch the train and those thoughts pass by – as a bystander or as if you're the countryside the train is traveling through. You don't have to get on the train...you can let it pass you by. These are just thoughts...they are not facts. They are not you, they are just mental events happening in your brain.

Of course, my evil twin still shows up every now and then and derails my train of thought toward an unexpected destination, (I'm only human)...but if I take a few moments to focus on my breathing and notice my thoughts and sensations Morgan Freeman isn't too far behind (I bet you can hear his voice right now too).

Exercise:

Sit quietly for a moment or two and think of some automatic negative thoughts you have about yourself i.e. I'm a crap driver, I'm no good at _____

Allow yourself to really focus on the experience of having that thought…. let it come up fully in your experience…notice how you feel physically and emotionally for about 20 seconds.

Now add these words or similar right before that automatic negative thought "I'm having the thought that I'm no good at _____." Try it for another 20 seconds.

Now add "That's interesting I'm having the thought (insert automatic negative thought)" for another few seconds.

Over the next few days try to notice these 'ANTS' and try this strategy again by saying to yourself 'that's interesting, I'm having the thought that I won't be able to breastfeed.'

Once you do this you are turning on activity in one part of your brain that begins to soothe the emotional part of your brain that is churning out these negative thoughts and feelings. You begin to become distanced from the thought and emotion and it's all a lot less personal.

WORRIED ABOUT PREGNANCY WEIGHT GAIN? EAT MINDFULLY

Food – it's on your mind from dawn 'til dusk. In pregnancy you're very conscious of what you eat. However most of us don't pay much attention to how we eat. If you're like most busy women you probably inhale your food on the go and half the time don't even remember really tasting it never mind savoring it. But remember the last time you were at a fancy (expensive) restaurant? I bet you tasted every morsel of that meal and savored every bite.

Mindful eating means you pay attention to your food, you breathe in the aromas and notice the flavors and textures. You'll become more aware of hunger and satiety cues, and start to understand how emotions such as stress can teleport you to that refrigerator door before you've even had a chance to ask yourself the question – "Am

I hungry – or am I bored, stressed etc." It means you start to slow down, sit down and savor your food, bite by bite. Pregnancy can be stressful for some women – especially if you're juggling a family and career. And we're more likely to overeat when we're stressed (ice cream anyone?). Stress is a trigger for many women to overeat because it signals the body to produce cortisol, a hormone that both increases high calorie food craving and fat retention.

Despite what you've heard pregnancy is not a time to eat for two (sleep for two is great advice). Pregnancy is not a time for crash diets. Excessive weight gain in pregnancy can bring with it potential complications for you and your baby. Mindful eating helps you to eat healthier, reduce stress and improve the health of your unborn baby – and without any feelings of deprivation. Elissa Epel, a researcher who studies stress and eating, ran a study (MAMA) which trained chronically stressed, pregnant women with high BMIs in the skills of mindful eating.

WHAT DID THE MOMS SAY?

They learned how to appreciate the taste and texture of food.

They could identify true hunger cues rather than eating out of stress or boredom.

They paid more attention to the sensation of being full so they ate less.

Mindful breathing exercises helped moms handle stress better.

They had lower weight gain in pregnancy.

BENEFITS FOR BABIES TOO

The research also suggested that the babies born to the mothers who went through the MAMAS program had healthier birth weights. Better birth weights translate into long-term health benefits too.

Unless you're eating while reading all this talk of food means your mind is probably heading toward the kitchen right now. But before you reach into the fridge - check in with yourself...are you truly hungry? I've had two kids I know better than to stand between a pregnant person and their fridge – it never ends well. Put a moment's pause between you and the fridge and just for a second think about what brought you there – stress or Snickers?

BIRTH STORY

Get Your Mojo Back

Myself and my partner, Frank, took part in Niamh's GentleBirth class in July in preparation for our daughter's birth in September. The majority of my pregnancy was filled with the usual horror stories and I want to share my (quite long!) story with you because it's the exact opposite, which is very rare to hear these days.

My guess date was 8th of September and although I believed she would come to meet us early, she didn't! I went for a routine checkup and I requested a sweep, something I was previously strongly against based on my research but my impatience was really getting the better of me.

Thursday 14th about 9 pm I started feeling the slightest surges. They were timing in at 1 minute long and 9 minutes apart. Because they were so bearable and focused in my lower back, I didn't want to believe it was finally the real deal. I had gotten my hopes up so many times and ended up disappointed. They were gradually getting closer together so I decided to get some sleep. I woke up at 5 am to no surges. I woke Frank up, had a good cry and went back to sleep. I was heartbroken. I woke up again about 9 am and my surges were there! 7 minutes apart and lasting 1 minute-this was definitely it! I stayed in bed with Frank, relaxing and breathing calmly with my hot water bottle. Time passed, contractions were getting closer together and stronger, but I was still so surprised at how bearable they were. At 2:45 pm my contractions were 5 minutes apart, 1 minute long and then my waters broke. They were colored with meconium so I immediately panicked, all the stories I had read about colored waters ended in a cesarean, and I had longed for a natural, drug-free birth my entire pregnancy. Tears filled my eyes, I lost my breathing mojo and intense pain flooded my body. Frank calmed me, reassured me, and I got my mojo back. Off we went to the hospital, eeeeek!

Arrived at the hospital about 3:30 pm and I was assessed as 2cm. I was hoping I'd be further along but whatever, it was what it was. I was admitted straight to the delivery suite at 4:15 pm. I was being constantly monitored, something I had not wanted, but because of the colored waters, it was necessary. As things progressed and got more intense, I decided to try Gas & Air. This totally didn't agree with me and I passed out. When I came around, I felt the strongest urge to push. The midwife checked me out and I was 10cm already and ready to go!! After 36 minutes of pushing, our daughter Millie was born at 17:54 pm weighing in at 7 lbs 15. The ecstasy just filled my body. I felt strong, empowered and unbelievably proud. Frank held me as I held our daughter and it was the most amazing moment of my life.

I had noted in my birth preferences that I wouldn't want an episiotomy unless it was completely necessary for the baby, I'm so thankful I did and they didn't carry one out. We were able to do delayed cord clamping, something which I was unsure about because we were unsure of how Millie would be when she was born, because of the meconium, but it was all fine!

She was placed on my chest for skin-to-skin, and she latched and fed straight away. Frank then took her and did skin-to-skin too, it was amazing!

Although I would've liked a natural 3rd stage, it ended up being managed with Syntocinon but it didn't have any negative effect on my overall experience! My total labor time from 2cm to Millie being here was just 2 hours 16 minutes and because I didn't have an epidural I could get up and shower, which was brilliant and exactly what I needed!

Throughout my pregnancy, I was stopped by complete strangers telling me how awful it was going to be and everyone I spoke to seemed to know someone who had the worst possible time. If I wasn't so excited and positive about giving birth, it would have really gotten me down. Nobody seems eager to tell their positive birth stories and I wasn't going to post this. It's almost judged as bragging but it's not bragging, it's empowering each other and letting each other know "Hey, you've got this!" It wasn't easy and it wasn't pain-free, it was difficult and tough even though it was so short. But it was also easily the most amazing and incredible experience of my life, I wouldn't change anything about it.

I would never have had the experience I had if I didn't attend Niamh's class and if I didn't have the overwhelming support that Frank gave me for my entire pregnancy and birthing experience. This is what made it so perfect.

"The instant of birth is exquisite. Pain and joy are one at this moment. Ever after, the dim recollection is so sweet that we speak to our children with a gratitude they never understand."
–Madeline Tiger–

HEALTH BEGINS BEFORE BIRTH

"How the mother holds the baby in her mind before birth affects the baby's future development"
–Dr. Catherine Monk–

Did you know your baby can hear, taste, experience, and even learn before he's born? But before you start playing French tapes to your bump, at this point the only thing your baby needs to know is how much he is loved. There have been significant advances in the study of how our babies are affected by our emotional state before birth. In an interesting piece of research several years ago, Dr. Michael Lieberman demonstrated that an unborn baby experiences stress (measured by his heart rate) each time his mother thinks of having a cigarette. Just the idea of having a cigarette is enough to upset the baby. Of course, the baby has no way of knowing his mother is smoking or thinking about it but his brain is sophisticated enough to associate the experience of her smoking with the unpleasant sensation it produces in him. Nurses and midwives often comment on how a baby's heart rate increases the more distressed a mom is in labor.

As this new science is only starting to hit the mainstream newsfeeds and out of context it can be a little (actually a lot) worrisome. New research suggests even moving house in the first trimester is associated with preterm and lower birth weight babies. Of course moving house isn't always something we can put off but having some strategies to manage the associated stress is very helpful. Fetal programming theorizes that environmental conditions during your baby's time before he's born increases or decreases his risk of health issues later in life such as obesity, Type 2 diabetes, autoimmune conditions and mental health issues such as ADHD.

What do I mean when I say environmental conditions? As your baby is floating blissfully in that warm pool of amniotic fluid his long-term health is influenced by factors such as your diet, chemicals you are exposed to (nothing new here) and stress (yikes!). It can even change how certain genes are switched on or off in your baby influencing not just your baby's health, but potentially your grandchildren's health too as these gene changes are handed down to future generations.... take a moment to let that sink in...then take a deep breath and read on.

▌STRESS IN PREGNANCY

By focusing on the things that make us happy in pregnancy we're allowing less room for stress. Think of ways you can crowd out stressful thoughts in pregnancy (this doesn't mean a daily visit to the Krispy Kreme drive thru).

In reality, some stress is actually good for you and your baby. It's necessary for growth and health. But ongoing chronic stress is a different matter and here's why. Your baby's brain develops according to the environment it's in - the signals it receives from your chemical messages (hormones). For 9 months your baby's brain is bathed in hormones dictated by your emotional state.... When you are feeling stressed those chemical messengers teach your baby's brain to grow differently. When your baby is continually bathed in stress hormones your baby's brain thinks "wow the outside world seems like a scary place – I need to prepare for survival and ensure the parts of my brain that will help me do that are on alert to protect myself from that scary place".

To keep it simple, the areas of the brain associated with survival grow larger and the areas of the brain associated with learning, language, and emotional regulation lose out as the blood flow is redirected to the 'survival' brain. As a society, I believe we need more babies born with brains that are built for WOW and wonder instead of worry and war. But before you go beating yourself up for taking the bait and arguing with the barista in Starbucks and accusing scientists of heaping on the mommy guilt here's the good news. We can't avoid all stress - as much as I would love to wrap you up in cotton wool and take you to a tropical island for 9 months that's not the answer. In fact, that could be incredibly stressful for someone who hates beach vacations (it's all about perceived stress). So, if we can't eliminate stress, are we then doomed to grow babies with less than optimal physical and mental health? Not at all – babies are incredibly resilient. In this emerging field of fetal programming, we're also learning how sensitive, responsive care of your baby AFTER birth can limit the effects of stress on your baby's brain. So YOU have to look after your own emotional health first to be that stress buffer for your newborn baby. (And don't worry you'll have plenty of opportunities to mess up your child over the next 18 years ;) every parent feels that way some of the time).

What I want you to take away from this book is learning how to change your response to that judgmental barista in Starbucks, your mother-in-law's stinging comments about your weight gain in pregnancy or how your newborn baby is sleeping (or not). Think of those events as an opportunity to practice skills to help you let those comments slip right off you like water off a duck's back. Now you know that whenever humanly possible your baby's brain can be marinating in the healthy hormones of oxytocin (love) and endorphins (happiness) and a lot less cortisol. The physical experience of stress and excitement are actually quite similar and you reframe the experience of stress in seconds and enjoy the challenge-response instead. You and only you have the ability to change how you respond to the stressors in your life – don't make stress another stick to beat yourself up with (as new moms, you'll have plenty of those) but rather allow the physical sensations of stress be your cue to refocus and redirect your attention and send some happy hormones to your baby.

Research alert - a recent study suggests that as little as 14 days of a 10-minute mindful acceptance practice is associated with a 50% reduction in stress hormone levels. Start today and you and your baby benefit immediately.

MAKING STRESS WORK FOR YOU

Stress can be perceived as a negative or a positive. Tiger Woods said, 'The challenge is hitting good golf shots when you have to...to do it when the nerves are fluttering, the heart pounding...the palms sweating...that's the thrill". It's not the amount of stress that's the problem it's how you interpret it. Shifting a stressful situation into a challenge response is known as cognitive restructuring or reframing. Take a few moments and think of a situation in your daily life that makes you feel anxious. Now describe this situation by

finishing the following sentence – "I hate the feeling of _____ " fill in the missing words....for me I'll say "I hate the feeling of...racing around getting the kids ready for school on a Monday" or "I hate the pressure of taking an exam when I haven't prepared for it." Now, let's think about this situation again; this time, however, I want you to restructure it in your head so you think about it differently....

"I love the challenge of getting the kids out the door on time on a Monday no matter how tired they are."

Try this and see how it changes your perception of stressful situations.

You are already an expert on visualization! If you worry (like most parents), then you have been practicing negative visualization for a long time and you're probably quite good at it. Constantly worrying about things going wrong during birth doubles the negative impact it has on you. If the dreaded event does actually happen, then you've suffered all those times you were worrying about it as well as at the actual event itself. And, if the worst doesn't happen (which is nearly always the case) and you haven't been worrying about it, then you haven't suffered at all.

BONDING WITH YOUR BABY BEFORE BIRTH

Many moms do not start to bond with their baby until almost mid-pregnancy, around that exciting time when your baby's first movements are felt. But from the moment you get that BFP you can begin connecting with your baby. Fascinating research shows that you start reacting to your baby's movements (your heart rate increases) before you are even consciously aware of those exciting movements. Much earlier than 20 weeks! Brain activity starts around six weeks of pregnancy, right around the time when you find out the good news. Focus on sending loving, positive messages to your baby. Of course, in this fast-paced world, it's impossible to avoid the majority of stresses in our lives, but we can learn to cope with them in healthier ways. One way is to take "baby bonding breaks" with your baby where you mindfully connect during the day (Cocoon of Calm is a beautiful short meditation for expectant moms in the App).

I'm not suggesting you have to force yourself to think happy thoughts all day but you can make sure you take the time to relax and use your imagination to send positive messages to your baby and choose better-feeling thoughts, for you and your baby.

Being aware of your unborn baby's consciousness and awareness can make the birth planning process easier. There's growing awareness that every choice made has potential positive or negative effects on your baby, making the right decision gets a whole lot easier. Now is the time you most affect your baby's future.

Think way into the future, to when your child is older... maybe starting or finishing college.

Now is the time to think about what gifts (the ones money can't buy) you want to give your unborn baby, and start doing the important work to ensure they have them later.

> "I wouldn't say I didn't feel any pain during my labor; the sensations were uncomfortable and unpleasant, and intense. But they weren't unbearable or unmanageable, or agonizing and, after breathing through each contraction, there was a lovely break before the next one came along." – GentleBirth Mom

HAPPINESS IS AN INSIDE JOB

So many of the stressors (and joys) in our lives are created internally and even more so in pregnancy. Without much effort, you can come up with a list of at least a few people in your life who have done you wrong ... the boyfriend who cheated on you as a teenager ... the woman in the supermarket yesterday who cut in line ... you get the picture. Those people have gone on with their lives and yet you're still stressing every time you think about them. When you think about these people, the emotions aren't pleasant and neither is your body's reaction to those thoughts. This exercise can help you build the 'muscle of compassion'. It doesn't happen overnight but it is well worth the practice and can change the emotional circuitry in the brain in only a few weeks. It's the equivalent of sending yourself and others a virtual hug (even those you don't particularly like). It's often referred to as a "Loving Kindness Meditation."

Of course, sending a virtual hug to someone whom you wish bodily harm to is a massive leap ... so we'll start with something easy and build on that.

Spend a few moments focusing on your breathing and getting settled.

Imagine sending loving thoughts (virtual hugs) to yourself using a simple mantra, such as, "May I be happy, may I be free from fear."

Now think of someone you are very fond of and send them the same intention: "May you be happy and healthy." It's easy to send loving intentions to those we appreciate.

For another moment or two, think of sending those same compassionate intentions toward a stranger: "May you be happy and healthy."

Finally, bring up that 'frenemy'... an old boyfriend, etc., someone who left you feeling salty and send them the same intention of happiness and health. This can be challenging the first few times ... those old habits of thought are still active ... your mind immediately wants to bring up that time when, etc., etc. ... it wants to activate those feelings of upset. Stay with it and send those intentions and wishes for wellbeing.

Even doing this exercise for 7 minutes has been shown to positively impact your emotional state.

A helpful strategy I like to use when someone is really getting under my skin is to find something in common with that annoying neighbor or judgy mother-in-law. It's easier to dislike people who aren't like us but if you can find something...anything in common with them the desire to smack them eases a little which of course turns down your stress response.

Try this example or come up with one that makes sense for you.

I travel quite a bit so this is one I get to practice quite a bit. There's a long line at the airport and you're late for your flight. The traveler in front of you is trying to go through the security checkpoint with various containers of liquids way above the rules and hasn't unpacked his laptop yet... standing there with a half mile gap between him and the next person (is your blood pressure rising yet?).

Remember when we perceive somebody as being similar to ourselves ("just like me"), we become much more likely to feel and act positively toward that person. You might mumble some choice words to yourself in that airport/ supermarket line before you settle into this exercise – we're not aiming for perfection – just a starting point to shorten your response of anger and lengthen your fuse a little.

"Just like me this person has experienced long annoying lines in airports."

"Just like me this person just wants to get home to his family"

"Just like me this person has had crappy days when nothing seems to go right."

These exercises are a lot harder to do when you're tired or hungry so gentleness with yourself is the key. Don't expect miracles. Keep the bar low. They all take practice but the more you do it the more your mental habits of automatically hating on the slow driver in front of you will change. You might still have the initial eye roll and sigh but the ongoing rage can be shortened. When other parents make comments about your birth preferences, your newborn baby's sleep habits, reading skills or your feeding choices this little practice comes in very handy.

STOP TECHNIQUE

Imagine you're late for work. As you speed down the freeway, someone cuts you off in traffic. Your stress levels increase significantly, your heart races, you shake as you honk the horn, and maybe you even speed up to shout at them or tailgate to "teach them a lesson." In that moment of anger, you've literally lost your mind. The logical, rational part of your brain has been hijacked by your perception of what just happened. An inner conversation is played over and over again as you continue your drive to work about how the other driver is irresponsible, selfish, dangerous, and shouldn't have a license, along with several expletives. You arrive at work angry and very stressed - your body and brain are on high alert, as you have mentally replayed a 2-second event for the last 15 minutes of your commute to work. Your boss makes a comment that you're late and you explode. Not a great start to the week.

Let's try it another way.

Imagine you're late for work. As you speed down the freeway, someone cuts you off in traffic. Your stress levels increase significantly, your heart races, you shake as you honk the horn, and maybe even speed up to shout at them or tailgate to "teach them a lesson."

Then you use the STOP Technique:

Stop the reaction.

Take a few breaths.

Observe the way you're feeling.

Pull back.......

Pull back - what's the bigger picture here? Take the helicopter view. Is there another way of looking at what just happened? Perhaps the other driver just got the bad news that his grandmother is in the hospital or his wife has just gone into labor with their twin baby girls and she's only at 30 weeks. Maybe he simply made an error of judgment - haven't we all made mistakes? Maybe he's just a crappy driver!

When you use this technique, you're no longer held hostage by your initial reaction to that driver ... or something your mother-in-law said or a colleague at work. You've learned how to change that reaction quickly. You are able to choose a new perspective; you've "reframed" that experience and your brain has, in turn, reduced that stress reaction and you arrive at work a lot less stressed and are able to have a rational discussion with your boss about why you were late. What a very different start to the day.

When you start to notice your thoughts and feelings, you can decide which ones really deserve your attention and which ones are going to get you wound up. The more you exercise that muscle of attention, the more you are physically growing certain areas of your brain - particularly the area associated with rational decision making. So you can make decisions about pregnancy, birth, and parenting based on facts rather than stress or fear.

As you'll see in the GentleBirth community there is an intentionally upbeat positive attitude – we always assume best-case scenario rather than worst.

SCIENCE ALERT: According to Hebb's law, when the same cells are activated in the same pattern repeatedly, they form a brain circuit - a network in the brain. But Hebb's law only works when special glue is used (the quantum Zeno effect) to hold the cells in place long enough so they "stick." The "glue" that builds your new and improved brain is created by focus and attention. Imagine you have a tiny electrician in your brain who follows your instructions, based on what you're focused on. This tiny electrician is rewiring and re-sculpting your brain every day and she spends extra time using this special glue wiring together connections on areas you spend the most time thinking about.

Is your electrician wiring your brain for a dramatic, fearful birth experience and a stressful painful start to breastfeeding? Or is she building out a whole new circuitry of connections of positive expectations as you retrain your brain for pregnancy and parenting wellbeing?

BRAIN BENEFITS OF MEDITATION IN PREGNANCY

More positive emotions.

Emotional resilience (the ability to 'bounce back' and react positively to stressful events).

Decreased fear and pain.

Less anxiety and depression.

Increased confidence.

Increased focus and concentration.

Reduces elevated blood pressure.

Reduces cortisol by 50% with mindful acceptance practice.

Facilitates positive changes in brain chemistry (neurotransmitters such as serotonin, melatonin).

Changes brain structure associated with memory.

Makes physiological changes associated with a slowing of the aging process (mindfulness is a lot cheaper than Botox!)

With all of these benefits why wouldn't you meditate? I know I'm probably getting annoying pushing this practice - it's not a silver bullet. Meditation doesn't stop crappy things from happening – but it can change how you think about the crappy things and that's a game changer.

MEET YOUR MENTAL MEERKAT

Check in with yourself a few times a day by simply stopping whatever you're doing for a moment or two and take a few breaths. Home is where the breath is.

When you feel anxiety, panic, or sudden anger, it's a "bottom-up" automatic reaction from a part of the brain that turns on the alarm bells (amygdala), whether the threat is real or imagined. This part of the brain is what I call your mental meerkat, always on the alert and often setting off panic in the whole colony when it mistakes a shadow for an eagle. We can tame and train the meerkat and stop that panic by taking the spotlight off that emotion for a few moments and putting your attention elsewhere. The breath is the best place to start. It's always with you and needs no special equipment.

TAMING YOUR MENTAL MEERKAT

In one study, after only 8 weeks, mindful attention was no longer necessary to consciously reduce the meerkat response; it became an automatic behavior. The fancy brain scientists call this a trait effect. So you can change your life and how you experience it in a few weeks by simply training the muscle of attention. Practicing the STOP technique is an easy way to tame and train your meerkat and put him to work for you rather than against you.

THE UPSTAIRS/DOWNSTAIRS BRAIN

Imagine your brain is an apartment block. You have an 'upstairs' brain and a 'downstairs' brain. Your upstairs brain on the higher floors is the part of your brain that's responsible for making informed decisions, planning, and rational thinking. Think of the upstairs brain being the wise, refined cultured professors who live upstairs in that apartment block.

On the lower floors of that apartment block is your downstairs brain. It's where the emotional center (fear/anxiety) lives. Think of it like the apartments where the rowdy college students live...and they are always looking for a party. Often the downstairs brain cries wolf and releases adrenaline into your body based on a thought that you had rather than a real threat. Thankfully we can train the upstairs brain (the wise professors) to calm down the noisy college students downstairs and bring you back to balance and calm. We do this with the intentional activities of focus, mindfulness, CBT, and sports psychology.

> "If a problem is fixable, if a situation is such that you can do something about it, then there is no need to worry. If it's not fixable, then there is no help in worrying. There is no benefit in worrying whatsoever."
>
> His Holiness the Dalai Lama

▌DAD'S EYE VIEW – BIRTH STORY

Hi all, firstly can I thank all of those involved in GentleBirth. My wife drew great encouragement from all of your support, guidance, and honesty about her pregnancy. It feels a little odd contributing to this as regardless of my genetic contribution to the situation, this has been a "100% Fiona Production" with all of the accolades deservingly going to her. I simply don't have the words to express my love, respect and overwhelming pride I have for my wonderful wife. She is amazing, women are amazing. FACT.

Having heard snippets of some of the birth stories and discussing differing options and opinions during the pregnancy I knew from early on I would like to contribute something as means of a payback for all we got from it. I would also hope some of my "dad Notes" might offer the lads a few pointers on how they could get involved.

Fiona has detailed everything in her birth story so I thought I might just add a few points to certain parts to help demonstrate where I could see gentle birth methods being an amazing help. If you are reading this without reading Fiona's it may be a bit odd.

Options...eh we have OPTIONS!!

Our little lady was not for turning, so when Fiona's waters broke I can honestly say my excitement was tinged with an element of anger, I did not want to have my wife have a section. Firstly for reasons of risk, recovery and the impact it would have on her post-delivery plans and secondly was that following two miscarriages I knew she had her sights set on a natural delivery to bring a long two years to a natural conclusion. If I was feeling this way I couldn't even imagine how it was playing out in her mind, well there was no changing things now so off to the hospital we went.

On examination we were told, yes, baby is breech, the inevitable meeting of our eyes, yes, we knew we were both excited but also resigned to what would come next. But no, given our unique circumstances, the team were happy for Fiona to try a natural delivery.

KABOOOOM went my brain, jaysus, I wasn't thinking of this... my entire mindset was on weeks of recovery after a cesarean, ensuring I was wearing a shirt so I could do the skin-to-skin if called upon and a million other things with 0% on a normal delivery. I turned to Fiona and I could see in that moment her whole direction had changed, I don't even think she realized that she did it but she flipped into GB mode. Her face relaxed, breathing regulated, and eyes closed... a few seconds or so passed and then she came back calm, collected and centered..."What do you think?"

Like everything in life, things don't go to plan and how well you can react is determined by the tools you have available. In the midst of an emotionally charged situation to be asked to make an instant decision on an even more emotionally charged topic to find an anchor of calm and clarity is priceless. It speaks volumes of my wife and her use of the GB tools she had developed.

The Ebb and Flow

Having been given the green light to labor subject to constant monitoring and a "just in case we need to do a section" epidural to be put in when things were "really kicking off" we, and by "we" I mean "She", set ourselves up to breathe this baby out. Sat astride a birthing ball attached to the monitoring machine Fiona began to focus, to center her mind on the task. I was behind her supporting her, keeping her topped up with water etc.

For the uninitiated (that means the lads) the monitoring machine records baby's heart rate and mothers contractions. The contractions appear like mountains of pain, high bad, low not as bad. I could see the waves of contractions on the screen as they built up, peaked, plateau and then recede. But these jagged peaks weren't being reflected in the calm woman in front of me. I could see the pain wash into her body, she rolled, arched, swayed, twisted with a beautiful elegance in what can only be described as a primeval dance. Back and forth Fiona leading the pain, directing it, owning it, allowing every wave to ebb and flow through her to be breathed out. The beauty of the dance harmonized by quiet moans. It was a sight to be seen, among the beeps of the machines, chatter of midwives and bustle of porters I was party to a picture of pure serenity. I don't do it justice, and I know if it had been me on the ball, regardless of my no-holds-barred tough-guy persona, I would not have been 1% of what Fiona had become. Women have a beauty all their own and none was more beautiful than my wife in those moments.

The Final Push

The agreement had been that, as soon as things were kicking off, an epidural was needed to cover off an emergency section if required, in hindsight this came a little too close to the end to be of any benefit to Fiona. During the installation of the catheter, Fiona had two major contractions; I suspect her having to change position from the ball had moved things along. Again she breathed them out like a complete trooper. It was then I noticed another great difference between this labor and the first; the GB techniques had preserved much more of her energy levels. At this stage of the first labor, Fiona was wiped and ended up having a snooze for about an hour through sheer exhaustion. This time around, she was bright, in control, focused and ready to go despite the rollercoaster of the previous hours. So with what felt like half the hospital entering the room, Fiona began to push. I was expecting a marathon event but, over the next 8 minutes, my stubborn daughter made her way into the world bum first. Given I was the most useless thing in the room at that stage I was able to observe the whole thing, pretty magical. The room was still and calm, with the laid-back doctors having to be reminded to catch the baby as the midwives aren't covered for breech deliveries. With the minimum of fuss, out popped Faela. Bum and back, then the legs flopped down and the rest nearly all at once. My family was complete... the next adventure was a GO.

All I can say is thank you GentleBirth for what you gave to my family.

SO as I said I thought it might be of benefit for me to put down a blokes side of the event and offer some tips for other dads to be, ladies this is in "Bloke" so if you don't understand anything just ask himself to translate

Notes for Future Dads:

- Don't be a bloke (dude) about this, we get off pretty lightly on the whole let's-have-kids thing, so leave the old "sure I'm more worried about wettin' the baby's head" clichés behind and get stuck into the whole event, it's totally worth it.

- If your better half decides to go down the GentleBirth or similar route, take it from me, it's not just another of her mental pregnancy things like mayonnaise on popcorn. It's a real thing that works, don't just brush it off – get on board. Listen to the audio, have a look on YouTube, check out the website. It couldn't be easier, ass+seat+internet=prepared.

- Understand the birth plan and what each item means, who will be involved and when you need to articulate these things. You will be the voice of **your** family during labor; you need to know what to say and what you are being asked. Again we aren't the ones dealing with extreme pain, so making sure all around you are fully clued in on your partner's plans, be it plan A, B, C ....Z. If we can remember seven different drinks when we are ordering a round of drinks at 2 am remembering a few facts will be a breeze.

- Ask questions about everything; not only will it give you great understanding, it will be good practice for when baby hits about 3 and EVERY sentence is followed up by "but WHY??". I'm sure if your better half asked you to explain the finer details of pregnancy, labor, etc., most of us wouldn't get anywhere close to top marks. Knowledge is key, what goes where, what the other does, you get that if this happens and on and on. You will regret playing the hapless bloke card who is just there by default, so don't do it.

- If you can get the above sorted then you are laughing, you are about 80% of the way to "Birth Partner of the Year"... (I'll be killed for that one).

- During the event remember the plan, be positive, supportive, and watch for the small details. What's comfortable, what's not. Keep your eyes open; always be considering what will she need next. Be it a cool cloth for her neck, some ice chips or even just wiping her face...her comfort is priceless.

- I spent about half of this labor just keeping the fitness ball from shooting out from underneath Fiona as she rocked forward and back. Remember, you are the rhythm section to your partner/s lead guitar. Be her rock, support her, take the strain, and always be positive. Reaffirm her choices, her strength, her abilities, comfort and caress her.
- One thing I will say on the talking is, for us less is more, I said no more than a handful of things to Fiona over the six hours. My theory on it was that she didn't want me cluttering up her mind as she focused. It's a bit like Jonny Sexton as he goes through his kicking routine, he has the crowd zoned out, he is one with the ball. The last thing Jonny wants is Paul O'Connell shouting at him "Go on Jonny, sure you are only brilliant, great fella, kick lumps out of it, I know you are totally going to slot this one over, you show them...." Less is more; know what to say and when to say it. Remember, as with every moment of the last nine months, regardless of the facts you are wrong, act accordingly.
- Enjoy it for yourself, remember you are 50/50 on this little person, soak it up, it's amazing. Don't have one second of doubt; you will be a great dad.

    PS. For those going to Holles Street, there is only one bloke's toilet (and I mean literally one toilet cubicle) on the ground floor for all of us. Make sure you take a note of its location near the admittance office, as at some stage, you will have to make a dash for it. It also serves to remind us how unimportant in the obstetrics world we truly are. You have been warned.

GET YOUR BRAIN OUT OF THE ANXIETY FAST LANE

As you know pregnancy brings with it an avalanche of information, worries about finances, doubts about how you'll cope and don't forget the never-ending conflicting advice from well-meaning friends and family. Throw some raging hormones into the mix and a demanding job and even the most centered mom can end up feeling anxious and overwhelmed. What can you do to calm the waves of pregnancy anxiety during the workday? Follow these simple mindfulness tips to feel calmer and more focused as you grow your career AND your baby.

- Be grateful – as soon as you wake up and before your brain takes off on autopilot to worryland take a moment to appreciate someone or something in your life. When your mind wanders bring it gently back to gratitude.
- Brush your teeth mindfully – pay attention to how your body feels... how your jaw moves...how the toothpaste tastes – do you look relaxed or rabid?
- Taste your food – breathe in the aroma instead of inhaling your meals.
- Remind yourself that right now in this moment everything is ok. The mind loves to race off to worst-case scenario and it's rarely the case. It's simply a habit of thought.
- During your commute pay attention to your breathing...is it deep or shallow? Turn the radio off for a while – allow yourself to rest in the silence.
- Slow down – as you walk to your place of work notice the trees, the cracks in the pavement, the temperature of the air.
- When you feel stressed – ask yourself where are your feet? (Simply redirecting your focus out of your head into your body helps enormously if a panic attack is looming).
- Take a walk at lunchtime – how does your body feel as your pregnant hips sway. What areas of your body are tense...what areas are soft.
- Connect with your baby – in the privacy of your own mind even in the busiest office you can have a private meeting with your baby - imagine holding your baby, counting

those tiny toes.......watching them take their first steps, hearing their first words.

- Be your best friend – not your worst enemy. Speak to yourself kindly, treat your pregnant body kindly you are growing a human being - how amazing is that!
- Repeat steps 1 - 10 every day.

"Birth takes a woman's deepest fears about herself and shows her that she is stronger than them."
–Unknown–

Two Questions to Catch Stressful Thoughts

Question 1 - What is my brain telling me right now?

Question 2 - Is it helpful?

When you do this you're acknowledging that the negative thoughts are not "you" they're your brain trying to be a 'fortune telling' machine. Those thoughts are just mental events. <u>You</u> didn't say "I'm a crap mom" your brain did. You're creating a tiny gap between you and the thought. And you can use that bit of distance to question the thought.

But often you'll question the thought and that negative narrator will come back with, "But it's <u>true</u>. I am a crap mom. Everyone else is better at this."

We could sit here with me trying to convince you that it's not true and you're an amazing mom and you disagreeing with me, but here's the thing: It doesn't matter what the thought is and if it's actually true or not; what really matters is the question "Is it useful?"

I don't care.

Is telling yourself that you have no pain tolerance, won't be able to breastfeed, etc., going to help you do the things that improve your pain tolerance or make breastfeeding more likely? Nope.

When you have that thought does it inspire you? Does it motivate you to practice your comfort measures or read everything you can about breastfeeding?

Step back and say, "Hmmm I notice I'm having the thought that _____."

Or "I'm having a mental event about _____."

That gives you a little distance. It holds the thought up to the cold light of day and lets you see it for what it is – a mental event – it's not you, it's a product of that grey and white organ above your eyeballs.

How is continuing those thoughts going to contribute to your positive birth? Are those thoughts going to make a positive birth and parenting experience more or less likely?

Once you've done this you can make a decision based on what's really relevant in your birth/parenting plans not your fears or worries.

LEARN HOW TO WORRY WELL

You can approach your baby's birth in several ways - put your head in the sand (denial), chronically worry and panic about every ache, symptom, and sign you have throughout your pregnancy, or learn how to "worry well" (Dr. Rossman). Most of us don't actively practice positive visualization in our day-to-day lives but worry IS visualization - just the unhelpful kind, and as I said earlier you're already good at it! Let's see how we can make worry work for you instead of against you.

MOTIVATIONAL WORRY

Motivational worry can be your friend - it's the "good" kind of worry. Perhaps today you're worried about coping with a new baby. Is that a reasonable worry for a first time mom or a mom with five young children at home?

Yes, absolutely! These kinds of worries have an important function for a mom-to-be - they are motivational. They drive you to action to find a solution and, once the appropriate action has been taken, the worry is resolved. In this scenario, finding out where your local mom and baby group is will reduce this worry. Or investigate hiring a postpartum doula to support you in those early weeks or enlist help from family/friends.

RUNAWAY WORRY

The most unhelpful kind of worry is one that keeps you in a constant state of fear and anxiety. It's usually about something that's out of your control and, because it's associated with the emotion of fear, it can become a habit of thought quite quickly due to the intense emotions associated with it. Becoming a parent brings with it significant life changes. Catastrophizing occurs when we look to the future and focus on all the things that could possibly go wrong. We then create a reality around those thoughts (e.g. "I know I won't be able to cope because..."). It's already a done deal. Buying into these kinds of worries (catastrophizing) is like giving up before you've even started. You feel like you've failed before you even begin. So you make excuses because you feel it's all going to go wrong anyway and there's nothing you can do. You feel powerless. You are buying into the belief without questioning your thoughts that you are destined to be a "terrible mother," or you'll be screaming for the epidural, or doomed not to breastfeed because your mom didn't.

PUTTING THE BRAKES ON A RUNAWAY WORRY

The first step to dealing with this kind of worry is to recognize when you're doing it. That feeling in the pit of your stomach will clue you in. It's helpful to keep in mind again that you are not your brain you are not your thoughts. Remind yourself that this is just a circuit in your brain that is misfiring and, as you do your daily-recommended brain training in the App, you are actively changing those circuits by using this program every day. This old wiring was installed when you were younger and didn't have the insight into how your brain works. When you find yourself ruminating over a particular worry ask yourself:

> Is what I'm thinking about right now rewiring my brain in a positive way or am I keeping those old circuits glued together?
>
> Is what I'm thinking about right now making me more excited about my baby's birth or more anxious?

It's literally a no-brainer! Change the channel! Each time you change your focus of attention you rewire the brain. When you focus you turn down the electrical activity in other parts of your brain. Make your brain work for you.

Try this exercise: Write out the list of current worries you have and list the things you can do to resolve them. If there are worries that you can't resolve, is there a way you can reframe them to find something positive or can you learn to accept them in your life and make peace with them?

Don't take your thoughts (or anyone else's) so personally; remind yourself that you just have a malfunctioning brain circuit running.

As the structure of your amazing brain begins to change with these exercises, the changes are accelerated by focused sustained attention - it's like a spotlight. This kind of focused attention is a form of mindfulness and it takes practice. You decide where to put that spotlight!

▌DISTORTED THINKING

Your brain is sending you distorted messages all day long through your negative self-talk: "I won't cope with labor" & "What if I'm not a good mom?"

Your affirmations can be a very helpful tool to focus your mind - your mental meerkat (amygdala) gets very excited by negative self-talk and negative imagery and releases stress hormones.

Who is controlling your emotional and mental spotlight today? Your obstetrician? Your midwife? Your mother-in-law? The stranger who cut you off in traffic this morning? Your defiant toddler? Or you? When you learn how to refocus your emotional and mental spotlight onto your reactions, you'll be a better parent and a better partner and you will reap the benefits of better health - mentally and physically.

A simple way to keep you focused and to challenge automatic thoughts is to:

- Check it – what are you focused on right now?
- Challenge it – thoughts are not facts – is this true?
- Change it – move your focus to something that makes you feel good.

Even 8 minutes a day practicing these techniques grows new neural structure. Think 10-minute abs - but for the muscle of attention in the brain for a better pregnancy and birth.

So, as you start to dip into the new practice of paying attention (mindfulness) and start to use these techniques more frequently, you're feeding your fears less and you're creating stronger brain connections for a positive birth. The less you feed the fears, the slower that electrical wiring works until it withers away and dies off. Remember that the initial feeling or thought is just a reflex that you have no control over but, when you realize you're having a mental meerkat moment, you can take action and redirect your focus and STOP the meerkat.

In a nutshell: **You Are Not Your Brain**

> Is what I'm focusing on creating positive birth/ parenting brain circuitry or reinforcing the old unhealthy one - or, in GentleBirth speak, is what I'm thinking about now making me more excited or more anxious about my baby's birth?

Being more aware and changing unhelpful thoughts is DIY remodeling of your brain for a better birth and better health. Jeffrey Schwartz's book, You Are Not Your Brain, includes some very useful tips for challenging unhelpful, stressful thoughts during your pregnancy.

Step 1: Re-label the negative thought - call it what it is, a brain cell misfiring (dodgy wiring). Your brain is running an old program that old neural circuit is firing off the one that keeps telling you that birth has to be very difficult ...

that the other moms know what they're doing. It's just that old habit of thought that had lots of that "special" glue keeping it together (until now).

Step 2: Reframe - It's the brain, not me (don't take the thoughts personally) - this calms down your mental meerkat so you can choose a more positive and enjoyable response.

Step 3: Deliberate Refocus. Take your attention to your breathing. Change the channel, go for a walk, use your brain training, and choose a healthy response.

THE ABCS OF CBT

Cognitive behavior therapy is one of the few forms of psychotherapy and self-help that has been scientifically tested and found to be very effective for moms experiencing anxiety, prenatal or postnatal depression. Cognitive behavior therapy helps us challenge our thoughts, which ultimately changes how we feel and how we react. Negative thoughts are like bullies and, like all bullies there are some tried and true ways to deal with them. Recent research suggests that combining mindfulness practices and CBT can reduce the rate of depression relapse significantly.

THE BULLIES THAT LIVE IN YOUR BRAIN

A wonderful midwife, friend, and psychologist, Rosemary, shared with me her metaphor for negative thinking in pregnancy using CBT. "They are like bullies in the playground. Imagine a bully coming up to you and saying you're an idiot. There are several ways that you can respond."

Accept what the bully says (you didn't do well on that assignment today so the bully must be right). "I must be really stupid." With this reaction, the bully will come back again and again.

Challenge the bully. "That's not true - I did really well on all of my other tests and I've been nominated to run the school science fair this year." The bully is less likely to come back and bother you again.

Ignore the bully and go hang out with your friends. The bully has lost her power.

Birth bullies are those unhelpful and often mean-spirited thoughts many women have about themselves. They often appear in the form of self-denigration:

Do any of these sound familiar to you?

"I'd like to try for a natural birth but, knowing me, I'll be the one screaming for the epidural."

"Everyone else seems to be coping - maybe I'm just not cut out for motherhood."

"What if I don't have enough milk?"

OTHER WAYS TO DECREASE YOUR INTERACTIONS WITH "BRAIN BULLIES"

Challenge Them Emotionally

Be compassionate - what would you say to a friend if she was very worried about coping with labor or breastfeeding her baby?

What would you say to your daughter?

List all the things going well in your pregnancy or your life right now. Find something in your life you are grateful for.

What affirmation would be useful now?

Challenging the Brain Bullies Rationally

First things first: Take your attention to something else that makes you feel better so you can think rationally. Challenging the birth bullies when you're upset or stressed is difficult because the rational thinking part of your brain has been turned off.

Step 1 - Test the validity of the thought - is it 100% true all of the time? Are there any other women in the world who have coped well with labor? Is birth difficult and long for everyone?

Step 2 - What evidence is there to show this is true all of the time?

Do all women find birth/breastfeeding/parenting difficult all of the time?

Step 3 - When you are not feeling upset do you think about the situation differently?

Be louder than those thoughts in your head!

Byron Katie is an expert on fear resolution and helps thousands of people from all over the world challenge their thoughts about the world. The following exercise is based on Byron's life-changing process, known as "The Work."

Your thoughts about birth are not the problem...it's only when you believe them that it becomes an issue.

Try to come up with some stress-free reasons to keep thinking the way you currently do about birth and breastfeeding.

Do these thoughts about birth make you feel better or worse? By focusing on fears about birth you are choosing to feel worse.

Who would you be without that story (the scary thoughts about birth)?

- Ask yourself - is it true?
- Can you absolutely know that it's true?
- How do you react when you think those thoughts? (Give specific examples - how you treat yourself and others).
- Who would you be without that thought? Imagine yourself without those fears of birth...how do you feel?

Visit **TheWork.com** for more information.

What if your mind was incapable of thinking the thought "scary birth"? What would that look like for you? I imagine you would enjoy every day of your pregnancy and know that in a few weeks or months you are going to be holding your baby. You would look at birth neutrally or positively because you know that you can challenge those birth bullies.

See yourself without that story? How do you look? How do you feel? Are those thoughts of labor real or are they just imagined?

Can you say without a doubt that they are guaranteed?

For most women giving birth is a normal physiological process. Our attitudes and emotions interfere with the ability to have a positive birth so much more than we realize. A 'successful' GentleBirth isn't about pain-free birth three-hour labor; a "successful" GentleBirth comes from the peace of mind of knowing you did your very best to have the safest and most gentle birth possible for you and your baby. You stacked the odds in your favor. So, in the rare event that something unexpected does come up on the day and medication makes sense or intervention becomes necessary, there's no guilt. You did everything you possibly could to have the best birth possible for you and your baby.

We don't know what the future holds for any of us, so why not act as if you're going to have a positive birth instead of a terrible one. In GentleBirth we choose to focus on the best-case scenario every day instead of the worst-case. It's always a choice.

> Sometimes our habits of thought focus on what's not going right for us.
>
> Today try to notice what's not wrong.
>
> Shift your mindset to appreciation instead.

▌PREPARING FOR THE BIRTHING OLYMPICS

I always enjoy how dads sit up and take notice in the class when we start talking about the psychological strategies of their favorite football team. We're speaking their language! There's an incredible amount of research supporting the recommendations. Sports psychology principles help you and your partner prepare for birth in the following ways:

- Mental imagery and mental practice
- The practice of intentional focus
- Goal setting
- Motivation and positive self-talk

Let's talk about the value of mental imagery and mental practice. Rehearsing your birth 'mind movie' is an integral part of birth preparation but so many parents are experts in visualizing the kind of birth they DON'T want. When I speak to mothers about the kind of birth they'd like if they could write their birth story today as if it's already happened they'd happily rhyme off a list of things they don't want – unbearable pain, feeling out of control, an episiotomy, the cesarean, sutures. But ask them to shift that spotlight of focus to the kind of birth they DO want and I'm usually met with blank stares... most have never considered that their birth experience could be positive, that it might be incredible, it could be calm, it could be manageable, it could be short etc. Years ago an obstetrician commented to me how interesting it was that first-time

GentleBirth moms tend to act as if it's not their first baby – they act as if they've done it before...which of course they have. A GentleBirth mom who has been rehearsing her baby's birth over and over in a way that excites and uplifts her behaves quite differently on the big day. Remember, the brain cannot tell the difference between something you're experiencing right now and something you're vividly imagining, so each time you rehearse your baby's birth (works for breastfeeding too) your brain thinks this is happening now and either turns on the stress response, the challenge-response, or the relaxation response.

YOUR BRAIN THINKS IT CAN TELL THE FUTURE

What I mean by that is your brain is a guessing machine. It's a little lazy that way – it scans in your memories for experiences that it thinks are similar. It is bombarded by millions of signals coming from your internal experience (your back aches, you're thirsty) and the external experience of all of your senses. Information from our senses is altered by what we expect to experience and what we focus on. Research in neuroscience has suggested that you don't see the color of the sky but you anticipate its blueness and use your sense of vision to adjust this prediction (remember the white and gold (or was it blue and black dress) that sparked a Facebook debate in 2015?

The world is a constantly changing uncertain place so for survival, the brain jumps ahead to make assumptions based on previous experiences. The brain wants to avoid surprises and will use your expectations, previous experiences, and beliefs to predict the future - or the human race won't survive to pass on our genes. We're unconsciously always predicting what will happen next and you already have a 'mental model' an expectation about what birth is all about and when things don't happen according to our expectations the brain tends to explain away anything that doesn't line up with those expectations. But is that model based on fact or expectations, beliefs, and assumptions?

Take this example from interrogation experts;

Imagine a detective entering into an interrogation with the belief that the suspect is guilty of the crime under investigation. Based on that belief the detective may then predict that the person will likely lie about their involvement in the crime. Therefore, anything the person says or does will be filtered through this lens by the detective's brain and look for things to support that prediction. This issue is compounded when the detective has misinformation about what deceptive behavior looks like, so if the person shifts in their chair or scratches the back of their neck they may conclude it is due to them lying.

If there is evidence or testimony from another source that comes to light which lends credibility to the suspect's account, that information may be overlooked or discounted and may be explained away by the detective. For instance, testimony from a friend who states that the suspect was with them at the time of the incident and therefore could not be involved may be viewed with suspicion and doubt, leading the detective to conclude that the two of them have conspired to line up their stories.

This is not only supported through psychology and cognitive science with the issue of confirmation bias, but also neuroscience which tracked the electrical activity within the human brain, so it is a psychological and biological issue as well.

Truthsleuth.com

What does that mean for you? Well if your 'previous' birth experience (i.e. the negative birth you've been mentally rehearsing) and combined with scary TV shows and birth stories then this is all your brain has to go on so it will jump to the conclusion that birth must be accompanied by terror, tearing, extreme stress and unrelenting pain so next stop is your body in panic mode once labor starts.

Note:

This is NOT about manifesting a birth experience based on The Secret.

MENTAL IMAGERY AND YOUR BIRTH REHEARSAL

The value of using mental imagery to rehearse events is recognized as a way to enhance performance in musicians and surgeons and can even be used to speed up the physical rehabilitation after a stroke. 'Be like water' – one of the most famous quotes of Bruce Lee. The metaphor of the ocean is a common way of describing our emotional state of mind. In the GentleBirth Birth Rehearsal, there is imagery of going within to the calm deep space below the waves where mom and baby can be together – even when the waves are crashing above. British marathon runner Paula Radcliffe visualized herself running up the final stretch of the race venue in London. As she said at the time, I try to imagine that I'm in the closing stages of the marathon in London ... I just visualize myself running up The Mall. The metaphor of the marathon is one that resonates with GentleBirth moms. I've taught triathletes, marathon runners, and rock climbers and they all use mental imagery as part of their event preparation and self-motivation when they reach that 'wall' (which you might face in labor). They have learned to draw on their inner resources so they can still put one foot in front of the other even when their body wants to stop...to keep taking that ONE step...and then next...staying in the moment and taking one step and one breath at a time. Psychologists use the term mental imagery to describe this process which we use every day. For example, if you close your eyes, you should be able to imagine where the windows are in your home (visual image), the sound of your partner's voice (an auditory image). We can get totally engrossed in mental imagery. Research by the British Transport Research Laboratory showed that listening to sport on the radio can affect drivers more than being drunk at the wheel. Even more fascinating is that during simulated driving scenarios, there were nearly 50 percent more incidents involving hard braking while motorists were listening to sports commentaries on the radio than when drivers were driving without the presence of distractions. Maybe some nice soothing music is the way to go!

The most important aspect of mental imagery is arousal control (e.g., you visualizing yourself feeling calm and focused during your baby's birth) and building self-confidence (visualizing yourself feeling confident and coping). Professional golfer Darren Clarke says "If you don't visualize then you allow other negative thoughts to enter your head." Not visualizing is almost like turning on Google Maps but not entering your destination into it. It can only work if you put the destination in. GentleBirth moms rehearse their births over and over again...seeing themselves on the day...coping well... staying focused...etc. Muhammad Ali talked about creating 'future history'. Prior to a fight, Ali would visualize himself progressing through the whole event and see himself winning and feel those emotions. He would immerse himself in his imagination and repeat the dress rehearsal in his mind over and over again. The mind cannot tell the difference between what's vividly imagined and what you're currently experiencing. The problem is that you have probably been mentally rehearsing the kind of birth you DON'T want. It's a habit of thought. Your visualization practice is more powerful when you can emotionally connect with the imagery... visualize your labor experience in 3D... see it... feel it, enjoy it... Vividly seeing yourself in labor being focused and strong... deeply feeling the calmness and focus on the day...enjoying the feeling of anticipation knowing the baby is on the way can be a daily practice that gets you psyched and excited about labor.

You've Got This!

FOCUS TRAINING

A large part of GentleBirth is about learning how to train your focus. According to sports psychologist Dr. Aidan Moran, focus is the ability to concentrate or pay attention to the task at hand while ignoring distractions and is a crucial prerequisite of successful performance in sport (and definitely an unmedicated birth). In our workshop, we do an exercise with partners to help them anticipate internal and external distractions and get them thinking about how they will facilitate maintaining that focus for you and help you to manage emotional arousal through the 'Switch' technique. Andy Roddick, U.S. tennis star, revealed that in his 2007 Wimbledon match that he avoided making eye contact with his opponent in case he might lose his concentration. Snooker player Mark Williams sang a song to himself silently to block out negative thoughts in 2003. Some moms find just repeating the affirmations or the mantra of "I can do anything for a minute" or "Open open open" works really well for them. It's important to note that a focused mind requires deliberate mental effort, intention, and practice. You have to train that muscle of focus rather than hope it'll just happen on the day. Irish rugby player Ronan O'Gara says, "I have to be focused. I have to do my mental preparation. I have to feel that I'm ready". You are optimally focused when you are in the moment and staying with sensations such as "I'm breathing up with this surge...my body is moving gently."

Things get tricky with focus when you start to think about things that are outside of your control...such as 'how long is this going to take'? Focus is never really lost – it's just moved somewhere else. Where is your spotlight of focus today? The GentleBirth mantra of calm, confident, and in control isn't about controlling birth (although there are some areas you do have control over)...it's about controlling your focus, attitude, and responses to changes that may occur and paradoxically at a specific point in labor – giving up that control to your body and baby.

WHICH WOLF ARE YOU FEEDING?

You may be familiar with this story – an old Cherokee Indian was talking to his grandson about a battle that goes on inside all of us. He said, "My son, the battle is between two 'wolves' inside us all. One is bad. It is anger, greed, arrogance, self-pity, guilt, resentment, lies, superiority, and ego.

"The other wolf is joy, love, hope, serenity, humility, kindness, and compassion. The grandson thought about it for a minute and then asked his grandfather: 'Which wolf wins the battle?" The old Cherokee simply replied, 'The one you feed.'"

This is such a simple but profound story. We have a choice; feed the Good Wolf and it will show up our habits, our self-talk, and our behavior positively. Or feed the Bad Wolf and see how that impacts your life. The crucial question for you to consider is "Which wolf are you feeding today?" Which wolf will bring you closer to a positive birth and your parenting goals?

Athletes talk to themselves all the time (so do mothers so get used to it) either silently or out loud when they train and compete. British Olympic athlete Paula Radcliffe always counts her steps silently to herself during races to keep her focus. As she explained, "when I count to 100 three times, it's a mile. It helps me to focus on the moment and not to think about how many miles I have to go. I concentrate on breathing and striding and I go within myself". Instructional self-talk (using specific cue words or phrases improves performance). There are two kinds of self-talk - instructional (I need to breathe slowly down to my baby, calm, confident and in control) and motivational – "I can do anything for a minute, I've got this, I feel strong." Motivational self-talk seems to be more effective for endurance activities and sometimes that's exactly what an unmedicated birth can be.

"Educating the mind without educating the heart is no education at all"
–Aristotle–

MENTAL GRIT

Developing mental toughness allows you to persevere through challenging circumstances and emerge without losing confidence. The following attributes are all key for mental toughness (I've narrowed them down specifically for birth and parenting).

- Having self-belief in your ability to have a positive birth and parenting experience
- Being able to recover from setbacks or wobbly moments
- Having a high amount of motivation and desire to have the most positive birth for you.
- Having the ability to calm and soothe yourself following uncontrollable events.
- Having the ability to overcome emotional and physical pain.
- Having the ability to remain fully focused even in the face of distraction (busy hospitals).
- The ability to switch your focus when necessary.

Mental toughness focuses on 3 Cs, too – commitment (how much work you put into preparing), control (the extent to which you can control certain elements, controlling the controllables), and challenge (the capacity to see unexpected events as a challenge rather than as a huge setback). Eventually, a 4th C was incorporated – confidence. Not too far off our mantra of calm, confident, and in control.

When it comes to motivation some people think that motivation is something that either you have or you haven't (and it always seems a bit harder to find on a Monday morning). Sports psychologists refer to intrinsic motivation - this is a personal goal (wanting to have an unmedicated birth for the challenge of the experience – to see how strong you can be). I've found this to be really evident with VBAC (vaginal birth after cesarean) moms. There's also extrinsic motivation – engaging in an activity as a means to an end but not for its own sake. For some moms, it's about wanting to prove to peers that they can birth unmedicated or to have a VBAC so they can lift their toddler after the new baby arrives. Most GentleBirth moms are intrinsically motivated – hopefully you're reading this book because you feel motivated to have the healthiest, most positive experience possible – not because it's a trendy thing to do or because your sister had an easy labor.

Take some time to think about your goals for the kind of birth you want and what is motivating you? Are your current levels of motivation enough? How can I help you grow that motivation to reach your goals?

Goal setting is extensively researched in sports psychology. Your goal must be specific, realistic but also feel challenging, they should be written down and it's a good idea to check back often to see how you are progressing. The biggest challenge of doing the practices discussed in this book aren't the exercises themselves it's deciding to make them a priority in your life. There's very little hard work involved in turning your phone to airplane mode, lying down comfortably and then pressing play. Can you spare those few moments every day for a happier healthier you (and baby)? Seems like a no brainer. You don't need to go anywhere, or put on special clothing but some moms just won't make that time. Fear of birth is a choice – you have an alternative, right here in your hands.

SPECIFICITY

When it comes to birth preparation we need a specific goal for practice for example –

Five days a week...I will spend 20 minutes practicing with the App

I will do one activity mindfully every day this week.

I will walk 20 minutes every day to improve my fitness in pregnancy.

PROXIMITY

Don't wait until you're 34 weeks to start your preparation. Do something small every day in the short term. The earlier you start the sooner you'll feel the benefits and your motivation will grow.

Goal focus – our focus is on a positive birth as defined by you – not unmedicated or vaginal. Every day you practice you are one step closer to your positive birth.

You've probably come across the SMART goals acronym:

Specific, Measurable, Action Related, Realistic and Timetabled.

The one I prefer to use is INSPIRED

Internalized
Nurturing
Specific
Planned
I (in your control)
R for reviewed regularly
E for energizing
D for documented (write it down!) - think it then ink it.

FOCUS YOUR MENTAL SPOTLIGHT FOR BIRTH

You must choose to focus - it doesn't just happen - you must make a conscious choice.

Focus on one surge at a time - mindfully in the present - keep your spotlight on this one surge - not the one coming or the one just passed. Stay in the moment.

You are focused when you are doing exactly what you're thinking, as in "breathing through this surge."

WTF – WHERE'S THE FOCUS?

Choose where you direct that spotlight. Focus can be regained quickly.

You don't "lose" your focus/concentration - you've just moved it somewhere else. Bring it back to your breath, a point on the ceiling, or slow counting.

Birth partners can help a mother keep her focus with gentle and supportive coaching to help her maintain focus when necessary.

Birth Partners:

- Encourage mom with short-term, attainable achievable goals such as :
- Let's stand for the next surge.
- Let's try the bath for 10 minutes.
- Follow my breathing for the next surge.
- Let's change position for the next one.

BIRTH IS A HEAD GAME

Sports psychologists call this the "head edge." Positive visualization and positive self-talk are well documented in research to improve performance.

By visualizing (mentally rehearsing) your birth in as much detail as possible, you are creating a dress rehearsal for your mind and setting the expectation that you will be calm and relaxed during labor. Athletes employ visualization as part of their training and professionals mentally rehearse presentations and speeches. So athletes see themselves winning the Olympic gold and the entrepreneur sees himself closing that million- dollar deal. SEE yourself at the hospital or at home with your midwife, FEEL how confident and relaxed you are. BE THERE NOW. Act as if it's already happened. The famous boxer Muhammad Ali called this technique making "future history."

Imagine you are making a film of your upcoming birth..... YOU are the director and producer; YOU decide who is in your movie; anything is possible in your movie, See yourself relaxing at home on the couch or standing in the kitchen or wherever you want to be. It's 10am on a bright Friday morning; it's your movie and you can decide what time your labor will start, what the weather outside will be like. See how excited you'll be when you call your partner to tell him/her it's time... you write the script!

Imagine in this movie how comfortable and relaxed you feel, the excited drive to the hospital and look, there's no traffic.... settling into your room. In the next scene, your partner is calling everyone to tell them your baby is coming today. See how wonderfully relaxed you are... The nurse tells you how great you are doing and she is surprised at how calm you are.

You welcome each sensation, knowing that you and your baby are going to meet very soon. Before you know it, you feel that irresistible urge to bear down. In your mind movie you'll notice how surprised and amazed your obstetrician is, etc., etc. Your baby is born at 3pm, only four hours after your first surge … you feel so good and your little girl is so calm and alert … you and your partner admire her little wrinkled fingers…and her bright alert eyes…

You feel fantastic and recover so quickly and, if you plan on nursing your baby, see your baby latching on perfectly, sense how confident you feel. Your body produces exactly the right amount of breast milk for your baby.

You recover so quickly, you just can't wait to get home and have your little bundle all to yourself. You rise to the challenge of parenthood easily and gracefully.

This is your mind movie - wire these brain connections more strongly every day by replaying this experience mentally over and over again.

Write and rewrite your birth story.

MORE MENTAL IMAGERY

Using visualization to prepare for birth is a simple and effective way to prepare for birth by reframing your perception of the birth process.

SURGES AS WAVES IN THE OCEAN

Each wave bringing you closer to your baby… carrying you along to your destination, where your baby is waiting for you or maybe you are traveling together with your baby to your destination.

Feel the waves surging stronger, they swell and rise until they crest and then they ebb away as you relax deeper.

The undulating waves stroke, soothe, and massage your baby nudging him down the short birth path to your arms.

THE TRAIN

If you have ever stood in a station waiting for a loved one to arrive, this imagery will be helpful for you. Each train approaches the station with great power and force and one of these trains is carrying your baby.

THE UPHILL CHALLENGE

Imagine cycling up a steep hill and freewheeling down the other side on the journey to meet your baby ... you don't know how many hills there will be, but you are energized as you feel the air on your face while you freewheel down the other side of each hill. You know that the steeper the hill, the more effectively your body is working and the closer you are getting to meeting your baby.

THE UNFOLDING FLOWER

The imagery of the flower opening is often accompanied by chuckles from many and it tends to reinforce the perception that visualization is only for moms who like tie-dye, gluten free and long flowing skirts. If this imagery appeals to you, this is one of the most powerful images you can use during birth, as your mind will make the connection to the opening cervix (it's difficult to imagine what a cervix even looks like!) The opening flower metaphor is a universal image for birth and combines the elements of wetness, unfolding, ease, and softness. Imagine standing in a beautiful garden by a still pond surrounded by your favorite flowers. It's early morning. You can feel the sun on your skin and there's a cool breeze - you can smell the fragrance of these beautiful dewy blossoms. As the sun moves higher in the sky, you see the delicate petals of the flowers opening one by one slowly and easily. You drop a pebble into the pond and you watch as mesmerizing ripples get bigger and bigger. As your body surges gently and easily with each petal opening more and more, your body also unfolds with ease and grace. The ripples in the pond get bigger and bigger as our body opens easily – like the rippling water. As you feel the urge to bear down, focus on the word "open"; even saying it to yourself silently relaxes the facial muscles, which also relaxes the pelvic floor. Have a picture of your favorite flower with you during birth; scenes of nature reduce pain sensations.

Be easy with yourself and try not to force the imagery - if these images don't resonate with you, find something that does. The more you can make the program your own, the more effective it will be for you.

BIRTH STORY

GentleBirth Twins

At 39 + 3 weeks pregnant with twins, my waters broke on the Wednesday around lunchtime and I had lots of surges that day and was so excited and nervous because it was FINALLY happening. (They had wanted to induce me 10 days earlier and I was getting a bit desperate for things to kick of naturally). The surges disappeared. That night my family were practically having a panic attack that I wasn't in hospital being monitored so I decided to ring the hospital and see what they said. Of course, they said to come straight in because of twins. I decided to wait till morning and have a decent night's sleep, as I knew I wouldn't sleep in hospital. We made our way the hour and a half to Limerick hospital on the Thursday morning and got there around noon. I told them my waters had just broken when I called them the night before as I wanted to buy myself a bit more time but they said I had to go on antibiotics anyway at that point. I was really upset because I was in hospital and I had such visions of laboring at home before heading in. They were starting to talk induction for that evening if I hadn't started myself and I was distraught as I almost knew I wouldn't go into labor because I was so stressed out. That evening I bought myself until the next morning and almost psyched myself up for it. I posted on this group page at 1:15 am just when they were giving me another dose of antibiotics and I then rolled over and calmed myself enough to sleep. Literally minutes after I had posted, I got my first surge and I struggled to pull myself out of bed it was so strong. I had another two surges leaning on the bed and then quickly realized that it was most definitely kicking off. It really threw me how strong they were as on my first birth of 20 hours they started so weak and took ages to really get going. I was SO excited I jumped out of bed and walked up the hall to the nurse's station where I was giggling with excitement that I was in labor. I had about another 30 minutes of surges walking the corridor and then the midwife said she thought things were moving really quick so she checked me and I was 5cm. I skipped down the hall to the labor ward and the midwives who greeted me said they had never seen a woman look so happy to be in labor. I was really buzzing. I had spent most of my pregnancy freaking out about birthing twins because there seemed to be so much hospital policy involved and I had always had visions of being strapped to the bed and having lots of arguments about epidurals and other interventions. I had two gorgeous midwives, one very experienced older lady and another younger one. Both were really supportive and wanted to do everything to let me have it how I wanted. A consultant came in and scanned me and twin 2 had flipped breech, so she said that she really wanted me to have the epidural and almost seemed to be insisting on it. When she turned away, the older midwife said I didn't need it and that she thought I would cope fine with a manual breech extraction anyway and that it was my choice. She made me feel so empowered and like I could do anything. I spent the whole labor at the side of the bed and they just held the monitors to my tummy rather than strapping them to me. The constant monitoring was one of my biggest fears and they just made it their business to do it in whatever position I wanted to be in. I was 8cm at 4:30 and Matt, my partner, was still not there. I was getting a bit nervous that he would miss it all. He arrived at 4:50 and I hopped up on the bed and lay on my side and birthed my first baby with one of the midwives. She was born at 5:04 head first. They scanned me quickly and twin 2 was lying transverse so the consultant got involved. He had to reach inside me and turn twin 2 and grab her legs. He was very quick and, with lots of gas and air, it was totally manageable. They made me do lots of pushing to get twin 2 out and she was born feet first at 5:11. All very quick. Two placentas followed and no stitches needed. Babies weighed 6 lb 2oz and 6 lb 8oz. Both babies straight onto my chest after a quick glance over by the pediatricians (who had been standing around on their iPhones, looking a bit bored). Both babies latched on and fed away. I came home on the Saturday morning as the help on the Friday night with breastfeeding/ someone just to hold a baby for 5 minutes was really awful. I had visions of my second birth being like my first, with hours of labor, so I had thought that I would listen to lots of music and have GentleBirth in my ears for the duration. I found that I was so excited to be in labor and it moved so quickly that listening to the cheesy pop music in the labor ward was more in tune with how I was feeling. One of the midwives put on some 'relaxing' music in the room at one stage and I got her to put on the radio again. The two midwives were really amazing and they kept saying they had never seen a woman so happy to be giving birth. It was a million miles away from how I thought it would be when I was pregnant; it was so much better and an incredible birth experience.

HEAD HACKING FOR BIRTH

The Clothes Maketh the ... (Birthing Woman)

What are you planning on wearing on the big day? New PJs...a hospital gown, a lucky t-shirt and sweatpants - or maybe nothing?

Did you know that what you wear influences your behavior and feelings? That wearing a white coat, believing it to belong to a doctor, increases your IQ (compared to a white coat you believe belongs to a painter)? New research describes these phenomena as "enclothed cognition." The clothes you wear put you into a different psychological state. A hospital gown puts you in the mind frame of being a "patient" putting on PJs for most people is associated with getting into bed. Think of a time a visitor called at your door unexpectedly and you were "caught" in your nightwear... did you feel confident or vulnerable and a little uncomfortable?

The July 2010 issue of Psychological Science profiled a German study showing that a good luck charm can help you improve your confidence in your own abilities. Professional athletes have known this for years. Tiger Woods always wears a red shirt on the last day of the tournament. Basketball legend Michael Jordan would wear his University of North Carolina shorts under his Chicago Bulls shorts to improve his performance. The Oakland Raiders wear black uniforms to help build an intimidating reputation in the NFL.

Other studies have also shown that women who dress in a more masculine fashion in interviews are more likely to be hired and teaching assistants who dress more formally are thought to be more intelligent than their more casually dressed work colleagues. So what we wear not only changes the way we see the world - it changes the way the world sees us. Think about what you'll wear on the big day to give yourself that birth "head edge."

BIRTH STORY

Flynn's Fabulous Arrival

I had a dream pregnancy, very little sickness, felt quite fit throughout, bar the odd cold and flu when I would have killed for something stronger than a paracetamol, but I really was very lucky. Obviously, like everyone, I had seen images of birthing in movies and on TV and was somewhat apprehensive about what it would be like for me. It doesn't help either that so many women feel they need to tell you a horror story about either the immense pain they or their friend's friend's cousin went through!

Well, I had a friend of a friend myself and she had taken on the services of a doula, a term I hadn't heard of at the time. Our mutual friend told me she was listening to relaxation CDs, was meeting with this doula, and was even considering bringing her into the labor ward instead of her husband. When she finally gave birth to her daughter, with her husband by her side I should add, I was told she listened to her CD during the labor and that, when the nurses told her it was time to push, she told them that it wasn't, popped her CD back on and a little while later told them she was ready. Kids weren't even on the horizon for us at that time but that set up struck a chord with me even then. The idea that you can be in labor and yet still be in control was not something depicted in the movies when it looks like a woman is being torn in two! So, when the time came for our baby, I looked up the services of Tracy Donegan and booked in for her weekend course.

I chose to go public for my maternity care and thought that, as we weren't spending there, it would be a good idea to fork out for this course and others, such as pregnancy yoga. The course isn't mad money at all but to be honest, even it were thousands it would be money well spent.

We both got a lot from the course, it was the first time we had both sat and talked and listened about labor - what to expect, etc. We watched women give birth using the GB method and that was an eye-opening experience. One woman was sat on the bed in the hospital looking peaceful, breathing deeply, her husband answered all the questions the nurses were asking and made sure the door was shut for her privacy, it was all just so relaxed. All of a sudden she just got up, her instinct was to birth leaning into the pillows and out popped the baby, even the midwife was shocked and had to rush to get her gloves on to help catch the new arrival! I kept that image with me a lot, as even though Tracy was convincing, you have to see it to believe it really.

So, armed with my MP3s and book, the GentleBirth advice was to listen to your tracks every night and then your subconscious mind will get itself and you prepared for a peaceful birth where you are calm, comfortable, and in control. Tracy suggested that you try and mix up the places you listen to it, not just in bed going to sleep every night but also when there's a bit of commotion going on, so you'll learn to zone out. I did my best with this but, to be honest, it was mostly every evening that I'd pop on the headphones. It used to help me to sleep and really began to change any negative thoughts I had about giving birth around and I had a very confident positive outlook toward the whole thing.

I had chosen midwife-led care through my hospital, which meant very few visits to the hospital; I literally only had to go in for scans, the rest of the time I went to a midwife clinic nearby home. Very handy, just a quick check of blood pressure, urine sample, and a measure of the bump and, unless you needed any further advice, which they were lovely at giving, you were on your way.

At around week 31, my baby began measuring ahead of schedule, so was the size they should approximately be at week 33. So they asked me to come back within two weeks as opposed to a month, just to see if it was a growth spurt that would even out. It was the same story at week 33 though, so from then on I was referred to the hospital to see a consultant, so they could scan the baby and monitor the progress from there. This was a bit of a bind because the hospital clinic was a lot busier than the midwife clinic but all for the good of the baby, eh!

At the hospital, while the care was fantastic, I was given ordinary scans and booked in for an ultrasound to best determine the weight and size of the child; From the first visit there was an air of caution exercised, that I was having a big baby and that either my dates were wrong or I might need to be induced or have a cesarean. All these were miles away from the gentle birth I was preparing myself for.

With all my preparation came an air of confidence about giving birth and I really felt I wanted to give it a go. I continued going for my weekly hospital check-ups and again and again they told me I was having a big baby, now over 8 lbs. and really their hope was I would go early. I went into overdrive hoping to bring on the labor, then would change my mind wanting to wait and let nature take its course, all the while this idea of a cesarean was looming over me.

I, and my brother and sister, were all born by cesarean section and in those days it was the norm to give a general anesthetic so my poor mom was out for days; now it's a fairly common procedure done using the epidural, so I'm not majorly against them, just as I say I wanted to give the birth a go naturally.

At 39 weeks, the consultant said the head wasn't engaged which suggested to him that, because of the size, it couldn't fit into my pelvis and he would recommend a cesarean, he immediately picked up and booked one for the following week. I left disappointed but, of course, thought whatever was best for the baby, I would go along with. The doctor said it could be a long laborious labor that could ultimately end in a cesarean, wouldn't it be best to just go straight to the cesarean.

Initially, I tried to be as positive as possible and was, of course, excited at the prospect of finally meeting my little one the following Thursday, but over the weekend I just began to change my mind. I was booked in for the section the day after my due date and I just felt that I'd like more time to go naturally. I rang the head of midwives and asked her if I could postpone and she changed the appointment from theater to an ordinary antenatal appointment. Again, I almost felt I was going against the clock to try and get the baby out naturally before being faced with a cesarean again.

My due date arrived and I had booked to have my hair done, I thought it best to stay as busy as possible and knew, either way, the baby was coming soon so the hairdressers would be a bit of a luxury I'd be without for some time. While in the chair, what I thought were Braxton Hicks practice pains I'd had before began. They got quite intense and at one point I thought I was going to ask the stylist to stop but I got through it, paid, and left. As I was in town and had a voucher for one of the department stores and fancied buying a nail polish you'd never spend money on unless you had a voucher, I ignored the dull surges and headed down. Picked up a bit of lunch and headed for home. These surges would then completely disappear, then return hours later, but I just went for a walk, chilled at home that night watching a DVD and having the odd sit and bounce on the birthing ball.

The following day, I had a bit of work to do, so I headed out to the company I visit weekly for voice-over work; even though I'd finished up for maternity leave from my main job, I kept this on as it's only an hour on a Thursday morning, though I had told them this would be my last time. As I finished, I headed to the restroom and discovered what I thought was the mucus plug. I really wasn't sure, as you get a lot of discharge at different stages of the pregnancy and there really aren't any photos of a bloody show in the books, I almost felt like keeping the bit of tissue to bring to my hospital appointment later that day but I resisted, flushed, and headed on.

Looking back now, I did rest a lot during those couple of days, more than normal. When an opportunity would arise I'd go back to bed and read my book or doze off. I think now I was conserving my energies.

As the pains were still coming and going, nothing more than a dull ache like period cramp, and I'd had this mucus. I was quite excited going back that afternoon to see the consultant that had booked my section. I was confident that he would examine me, say the head was engaged, and all would be well.

While he was very nice when we arrived, he was surprised to see us and when I explained how I felt it was rushed and I'd like more time past my due date to see if I could or would go naturally he was supportive enough and just said, "Well, let's examine you and reassess the situation."

Again, the head wasn't engaged and he said he would strongly recommend a cesarean. The one thing Tracy says when it comes to intervention by the hospital, whether it be induction, throughout the labor, or otherwise, is just to ask questions. Why are we doing this? What if we wait? Are there any alternatives? And most importantly, is the baby at risk? Once you've ascertained the answers to these, whatever the outcome, at least you feel in control of decisions being made about your birth, baby, and body.

The doctor was actually quite bleak that day and said things he hadn't the week before. One of the dangers he said was, that as the head wasn't engaged, the worry was that if my waters broke in a gush, as can happen to some women, the umbilical cord could come out first as the entrance was not blocked by the baby's head and then there was only a short time to get to the hospital. Missing this window could mean the child could be born with complications such as cerebral palsy or worse. Myself and my husband were shocked and I felt quite foolish, why was I insisting on a natural birth just because I'd done this course and listened to CDs which told me I could have this amazing birth experience? A cesarean was still a birth and wasn't the health of my child the most important thing?

I apologized, as did the doctor, who said perhaps he hadn't made all the details clear the week before, the clinic is very busy with only a short amount of time per person and anyway, we had said yes to the cesarean, allowed him to book it and I signed a consent form so he felt we understood and were on board. He attempted to book another for the following day, obviously having heard what he said I almost wanted one right there and then, but it was Thursday, they were fully booked the next day and there are no elective sections at the weekend, so he booked me in for the following Monday morning and said if I went into labor in the meantime, I was to get in to the hospital as quickly as I could.

I left a bit shell-shocked, but as I had asked the questions and been given the answers, I felt I now understood the why, I was in control, and I just kept repeating one of the GentleBirth affirmations to myself, "I will accept whatever path my birthing will take." I also called a very good friend of mine, who had two cesareans at the same hospital and had a lovely experience with each, no major issues with recovery afterwards, no problems with bonding or breastfeeding and, as she herself said, she never had to puff or pant and had her pelvic floor intact!

However, that night the dull pains returned. Again nothing mad, just something in the background; in fact pain is not an accurate description.

I was aware of them, was thinking, "Is this it?" but to be honest I was now worried about this umbilical cord issue and was annoyed at myself for wishing this on and trying a few techniques to bring on labor including aromatherapy oils, a ton of pineapple, and some yoga moves my teacher had given me. Again just a chilled night in front of the TV.

When the pains would go I would wish them back, when they'd come back I'd start to worry about the baby, but they continued to come and go throughout the next day. One of the suggestions to the partners from the course is to remember to keep the oxytocin levels high and the adrenaline low, this helps the mom to stay relaxed. It's suggested they do this by thinking romance, light candles, fill the bath, and watch a funny movie, so we spent the afternoon watching "Kick Ass" on the couch. I said I wanted to get a walk in, again switching in my mood; one minute I wanted to bring the birth on, the next I wanted to wait and have the safe cesarean. My husband works from home so, while he could be around, his phone can ring nonstop, so it was nearly 8:30 pm before he was ready to go for the walk and we said we'd watch another movie.

At this stage, I could feel myself getting agitated or restless, I kind of reminded myself of my cat when she had her kittens, in the hours beforehand she kind of paced around looking for a safe place to give birth. I was a bit like that looking back and was getting a little annoyed that my husband was just carrying on as normal but is just what I needed really. He asked if I wanted to walk to the video store and back which would have been at least an hour round trip, I snapped that he was being ridiculous, "This could be it, I could be in labor!" So we drove to the store - I was absolutely fine, the surges when they came felt a little sharp, but I really felt that if this was the start of labor, it was only the very start. We chose a movie, a comedy, and I said I'd wait in the car while he paid. Looking back it should have been more obvious, I really had to ease myself in and out of the car and breathe deeply but still it was totally manageable. So we drove up the beach, hubby helped me out of the car, and I hobbled over the road. I pointed to a life ring about 100 yards up the beach and suggested we walk to that and back, mad stuff really but I suppose it meant I was focused on something else and we were chatting away. The sun was setting and a woman went by on a horse taking him into the sea, I was taking it all in, but a little removed from it.

We came home and I had a bath, using the Love & Labor aromatherapy mix that Mary Tighe from BirthingMamas had sent me. Hubby came up the stairs to tell me he may need to work for an hour or two the following afternoon, I calmly told him that, while I wasn't 100% sure, I felt he should make alternative arrangements as we may be at the hospital.

We were probably at around 9:30 at this stage, though I wasn't really watching the clock. I was replying to a few texts, people checking in with me; I said to a few "don't think it will be long now" I then told Jonathan that it might be an idea to start putting my bags into the car, I still didn't think we were going anywhere soon but felt if these surges were going to get more intense over time then I'd sooner get any organization out of the way while I was up for it. I got dressed, into the nightdress I had bought for the labor ward, went to add leggings but tummy didn't like it. At this stage, while I was still happy enough, it was difficult to find somewhere to be comfortable. I didn't really want to sit on the birthing ball, though it had been helpful in the early stages sitting circling my hips, bouncing and rocking side to side, and I didn't want the bed or the couch. The toilet, oddly enough, felt quite safe, nice and dark, door, closed but not locked, hubby was never far away and he kept the lights dim everywhere.

Tracy had very kindly sent me a website about big babies written by women in similar situations to mine, told they were having "big babies" and that birth could be difficult. On it, one woman's birth story described how she found her contractions/surges were lasting about 10 seconds, so she would count along and when she got to 6 she knew that not only would it abate but she was also nearly there. I thought that sounded great and did it myself and it was very helpful. I told Jonathan what I was doing and that he should count along with me, though not out loud, just so I didn't need to be conscious of him looking at me and wondering if I was okay. He tried to tell me that they were actually lasting 18 seconds but psychologically I couldn't take that so insisted we stick with 10!

I got him to ring the hospital at that stage, we did a bit of timing of the surges and they seemed to be about a minute and a half apart lasting 10 or 18 seconds, depending on if you were going through them or watching! We didn't do this with military precision or anything, I was definitely a bit out of it or in the zone, as many of my friends who are mothers have described it. The midwife said that, if I could handle it, to stay where I was but feel free to come in at any time. They also suggested two paracetamol, which I couldn't even contemplate. It just sounded ridiculous, though perhaps they would have helped. I just stuck to my breathing.

At this stage, I said to Jonathan that if this wasn't labor and the surges were only going to get worse and go on for ages, then I thought I would get the epidural. I said, "Forget everything I've said before." He, of course, said whatever I wanted was fine with him. I suggested we drive to the hospital now. I was kind of pacing around or going to sit on the toilet and, while I still felt they were manageable, I worried that if the surges were to worsen that I wouldn't be able to sit or lie comfortably in the car for the drive into town to the hospital and once there I wouldn't be able to converse with the nursing staff and check in. I basically thought, let's get any organization out of the way so I can remain relaxed and focus on what's going on with my body.

Just as we were about to leave, my phone rang. Jonathan was pulling the car around to the front door. It was the hospital: they had just gotten my chart and saw I'd been booked for a cesarean section so asked me to come straight in. I was a bit breathless but was able to say we were on the way.

So we drove in. It was comfortable enough, though when a surge would come I would grip the handle and get Jonathan to drive really slowly as bumps on the road were a bit iffy but then after 10 it would pass and we would be chatting again, not idle chit chat now, but talking and I was thanking him for being so great, it was all good.

We got to the hospital, got parking very close to the door, and walked in. I had to stop for a quick 10 count on the way but that was grand. Jonathan checked us in with reception and the lady sent us to the assessment area.

A midwife came out and told us to wait in the waiting room. I didn't think I could handle other people, I knew it would make me self-conscious when a surge would come, so when Jonathan confirmed there were six other people in there I bailed into the toilet, locked the door & waited there. I prayed Jonathan would understand enough to come and get me when they were ready for me, rather than say, "She's in the toilet" and wait longer but I shouldn't have doubted him, that's exactly what he did.

I had a cold wet face cloth on the go from when we were at home and I found it very helpful. In the car, during a surge or during a break it was very soothing and relieving and gave you something else to focus on. So it was just me and face cloth in the toilet until I was called. I had a bit more mucus while in the toilet so when I got into the assessment room I told the nurse. She told me to hop up on the table for an examination. Again, I was very much in the zone, a little out of it, but feeling fine, I hardly even felt the examination. When the midwife told me I was 10cm dilated I was very surprised but delighted. That is the labor jackpot!

Next thing I know a wheelchair was brought in and I remember thinking, "Wheelchair good, not sure I could walk now" but again I was feeling fine. The lights in the assessment room were quite bright by my standards, I'm a bit of a vampire and like very dim lighting, so I put the facecloth over my eyes, a top move, as it kept me cool and calm and in my own little world. Hubby Jonathan just kept rotating the facecloth, getting water from the cooler on the corridor and I had one on my eyes and one on my chest; -I'd definitely recommend that they go into every labor ward bag. He also had a sports bottle of water, also kept cold and a straw - when you want a drink you only want a sip or few and don't really want to be handed a bottle, so that's another top tip.

I had the urge to bear down or push, so I was thinking to myself that I was going to shock them all, I'd already reached 10cm quite quickly or so it seemed and I thought, in moments this head is going to pop out. It wasn't quite like that, even though the surges remained manageable; about two hours passed with little change.

The head midwife that night came in then and suggested breaking my waters. Armed with the questions given to me by the GentleBirth course, I asked why are we doing this, is there an alternative, what if we wait, and is the baby ok? They were perfectly fine with these and it just let me feel that, whatever the next stage, at least I was in control and ultimately making the decisions. The midwife just explained that I had been at 10cm for a long time now and things should be moving on. I had spent some of my time in the labor room standing and wherever you go they put this sort of sanitary towel mat under you and there had been spots of liquid on that. I told her I thought my waters had already broken, but with my permission she just used her hand (to be honest I didn't even really feel it I was so in the zone) and the waters came rushing out which actually gave quite a bit of relief and I was like "Ah, so that's the waters breaking."

About an hour later (again I had no concept of time), I was starting to get a bit fed up, I wasn't in pain but I needed to know that there was a means to an end here, that at some stage there would be a crowning glory and a baby. My husband started to say he was hungry and so tea and toast was brought in to him and he ate that in the corner while I began to push (thank God I'd the facecloth clamped over my eyes so I couldn't see him dine, I was beginning to think of how hungry I was).

The head midwife came back in, she was very nice and I really trusted her but she was a bit of a military sergeant. I kind of needed it but every time she came back she'd be moving things along, so she ramped up my pushing. I told them I didn't want to put my chin to my chest but with their encouragement, (the toast muncher was also back by my side swapping facecloths and offering water sips) I began to push harder with their coaching. The midwife was saying "Come on, come on, come on, three long pushes, that's it," all that kind of thing and, to be honest, while I'm sure it helped I think I would have liked to keep the calmness I had earlier; but, as I said, I was as keen as they were to reach the finishing line.

The only time I felt a slight bit of pain was the stinging sensation as the head began to crown, but as I had done the perineal massage (not nearly as much as I should, I just did a few in a row over the last few days), I had felt the sensation before and was ready for it. But it did sting and to push into it was tricky, but my team of two midwives and hubby were very supportive and I knew baby was nearly here. They explained that they'd just give me a local anesthetic in case of a tear, again I didn't feel that injection or the little tear (I needed two stitches afterwards) but they asked me before they did everything. Next thing I know, the head was out and it's pretty much plain sailing from there. Before you know it, the baby pops out and, after a quick

bit of suction; they placed our son on my chest. I had a little boy, the birth I had wanted, a million miles from a section and all was great in the world. He was born at 4:31 am, weighing 9.5 lbs, we've called him Flynn and, while I am happy to enjoy our little man for now, I would go through the whole process again in a heartbeat.

FACIAL EXPRESSIONS - FAKE IT UNTIL YOU MAKE IT

"Sometimes your joy is the source of your smile, but sometimes your smile can be the source of your joy."
–Thich Nhat Hanh–

Your emotional state and even your facial expression play a significant role in how much pain you feel (and, believe it or not, you can change your brain's perception of pain just by smiling). Even if at the time you don't feel like smiling, just the act of smiling releases happy hormones, your natural pain relievers into the bloodstream muting pain. Smiling can relax the jaw, which is thought to relax the pelvic floor. Smiling is also contagious (as is stress).

The part of your brain that is responsible for smiling when happy or mimicking another's smile is in a part of the brain that has an unconscious automatic response. In a Swedish study, subjects were shown pictures of several emotions: joy, anger, fear, and surprise. When the picture of someone smiling was presented, the researchers asked the subjects to frown. Instead, they found that the facial expressions went directly to the imitation of what subjects saw. It took conscious effort to frown. So if you're smiling at someone, it's likely they can't help but smile back. If they don't, they're making a conscious effort not to.

A study at Australia's Flinders University found that that the pattern of brain activity triggered by looking at an emoticon smiley face is similar to when someone sees a real smiling human face.

New research also suggests that, when you frown during an unpleasant procedure, you're more likely to feel pain more intensely than those who do not. Those who exhibited negative expressions reported being in more pain than the other two groups. One scientist, Michael Lewis, plans to study the effect that Botox injections have on pain perception. "It's possible that people may feel less pain if they're unable to express it," he says. So are there fewer epidurals and more Botox in our future?

"It seems that many health professionals involved in antenatal care have not realized that one of their roles should be to protect the emotional state of pregnant women."
–Michael Odent, M.D.–

POWER POSITIONS

You've probably heard that being upright in active labor has lots of advantages - you're using gravity and movement to assist your baby as he spirals through the pelvis. Moms who labor upright also require less pain medication and babies have less fetal heart issues. But did you know that it's not just gravity that's at work here, but a mental state, too?

Think of how vulnerable and powerless you might feel when you're lying flat on your back (less than fully clothed) with strangers around you. Pause for a moment and notice how that thought makes you feel. Did you know that choosing a different position causes changes in your hormones and behavior?

Studies suggest that just by moving into a "high power" position (upright) you reduce cortisol (your stress response) and you increase the hormone testosterone, which gives you a boost in confidence and, in the words of one study, "increased feelings of power" - in just two minutes. By simply changing your physical posture, you are preparing your brain and body to handle the challenges of birth. Think of the Wonder Woman pose for inspiration.

Having a difficult conversation with your obstetrician or a co-worker? Nod and smile - nodding your head leads to more persuasion and smiling relaxes your body and increases humor responses. Try it with your partner the next time you're having a disagreement.

YOUR MEERKAT AND THE HEALTHCARE PROVIDER

Have you ever met someone you just didn't "gel" with? You've no reason that you can rationally think of why you shouldn't get along with this person. Yet you can't put your finger on what it is that bothers you about them, but something is off and you get a weird vibe.

Most staff will be very supportive on the day and really enjoy working with GentleBirth moms but, in the event that they are not "feeling the love" from your HCP, your birth partner can request a new nurse (without letting mom know) and this is why: If your nurse (or obstetrician) is smiling while reading your birth preferences but rolling her eyes "on the inside," the act of them suppressing that emotion can in fact raise your blood pressure. That little over-excitable friend, your mental meerkat, is very good at picking up other peoples unconscious "micro-expressions" and, due to the plasticity of your brain in pregnancy, expectant moms have a heightened ability for this 'super power' (possibly to protect themselves and their baby from a potential threat). So, while your HCP is trying to hide an emotion, your meerkat is firing off alert signals because her words are not in line with her initial micro-expression and your body is alerting you to this. If changing your midwife/obstetrician isn't an option, then use your other tools to calm down the meerkat to keep the oxytocin flowing. STOP and reframe - (maybe she's having a bad day or has been up all night with a teething baby).

THE SMELL OF FEAR

In pregnancy your sense of smell is heightened – and, during the birth process, it's bionic. Studies show that sweat from women who have watched a violent movie smells differently (more like aggression) than a neutral movie. Your mental meerkat has an exceptional sense of smell.

BRAIN HACKING WITH YOUR SENSE OF SMELL

The use of essential oils can be very helpful in keeping your meerkat in check on the big day to stop you picking up the wrong cues from your midwife. Imagining certain smells also works, as the brain reacts to a familiar imagined smell too. It's difficult to study brain changes in pregnant moms but, in studies of pregnant rats, there is a significant increase in the areas of the brain associated with smell (olfactory system), which plays a major role in bonding after birth. It changes significantly right after birth. Some medication, such as Syntometrine given to deliver the placenta, has been shown to impact this highly sensitive area so mom rats don't recognize their babies as well. We all know how the smell of our favorite food cooking can make our mouths water or how the smell of the sea air can transport us to our childhood by reminding us of wonderful days at the beach.

Evidence has shown that different essential oils can affect mood, blood pressure, perception of pain, and concentration. Japanese research found that machine operators' efficiency improved by 21% when the atmosphere was scented with lavender, by 33% when jasmine was used, and by 54% with lemon (even when the staff wasn't consciously aware of the scent).

Our sense of smell is extremely sensitive and it is possible to detect over 100,000 odors. When cells inside your nose capture odor molecules, they signal changes in the brain. That's why a smell can quickly influence your entire body (in a positive or negative way). Research even shows that vanilla reduces stress indicators in premature infants in NICU.

In 2000, the largest study on the use of aromatherapy in childbirth was published in the UK (Burns et al). Over 8,000 moms took part in the study in a busy UK teaching hospital. The goal was to examine whether aromatherapy improved mom's coping ability, reduced anxiety and perception of pain. Moms consistently rated the administration of aromatherapy positively. Lavender and frankincense were found to be most beneficial for reducing anxiety fear and pain in labor. A 2014 study also recommends lavender as an analgesic. Frankincense is wonderful for encouraging deep breathing (keeping the meerkat in check).

Peppermint was found to be most helpful for relieving nausea and vomiting during the birth process. It's also a great tool to have in your toolkit for focus and stamina clary sage was used to encourage surges in a slow labor.

Ways to use essential oils during birth:

- Labor pool
- Compress
- Diffuser
- Massage
- Droplet on pillow or clothing
- Inhalation over a steaming bowl

In one study, 635 moms applied lavender oil to their perineal area after birth. The women reported a distinct improvement between the third and fifth day. (The discomfort was the worst during this same time for women who did not use lavender).

The dosage of essential oils for use in labor should be no more than 1 - 2% for massage and 4% for baths; for new moms, a 2-3% blend can be used (4-5% in baths). All essential oils should be added to a base or carrier oil. For each 5ml of base oil, the number of drops added will be the same as the percentage blend required; e.g., for a 2% blend, two drops are needed.

For moms who have had a cesarean birth or perineal trauma, essential oils such as lavender and tea tree can be used in the bath as a preventative measure against wound infections. There is no evidence to suggest that using these oils in the bath affects stitches after a vaginal or cesarean birth.

For more information on the safe use of essential oils, talk to our aromatherapy experts in the GentleBirth Facebook group. Avoid using a diffuser close to the end of labor as your baby's sense of smell is heightened for bonding with you.

> **Note that in the UK 2000 study, aromatherapy was available to all moms regardless of obstetric history, with the exception of lavender oil for women who had asthma-related hay fever and mothers with multiple allergies only used chamomile.**

GENTLEBIRTH MOM

"I am so pleased I found out about GentleBirthing before the birth of my first child and that I used it again during my second labor. I was uncomfortable, similar to the worst period pains ever, but not to the point where at any time I felt I needed intervention or that I couldn't manage things. My only concern on my first labor was that the hospital seemed unprepared for how my labor progressed; it seemed that, because I wasn't screaming out in pain, I wasn't displaying the signs of labor as expected and as a result wasn't moved to the labor ward until I was fully dilated and therefore I missed the first strong contractions to push. However, the baby was out 40 minutes later.

"On my second labor, I missed the signs myself and arrived at the hospital just 40 minutes before the baby came out. I definitely don't think I have a high pain threshold, as I have asked about it, I believe it was through a self-belief that I could do it that I did it."

(This is why some medical staff call GentleBirthers 'sneaky' birthers).

RELAXATION AND BIRTH

Stop reading for a moment and think about how you feel when you are relaxed. Happy, confident, calm, full of energy, not worrying, you can cope with anything, life is good your blood pressure is normal, your breathing is relaxed.

So, by being relaxed in labor, you also have the benefits of all the wonderful side effects that come with it.

YOUR BODY'S RESPONSE TO FEAR AND ANXIETY

- Racing heart, panic, stress
- Shallow breathing
- Fight or flight response - blood is directed AWAY from the uterus and your baby, causing muscle spasms in the uterus
- Glucose release to fight/flee leaves mom tired

Sound familiar? If you replace the word uterus with heart in the above scenario, you'd be experiencing a heart attack! Our heart beats every day from early after conception until we die and it never hurts until its blood supply is reduced. Similarly, when oxygen-rich blood is redirected AWAY from our uterus (by the action of adrenaline and fight or flight), labor HURTS even more. But there's more to it than that. Adrenaline is only one part of the puzzle.

YOUR BODY'S RESPONSE TO RELAXATION

- Increased levels of oxytocin (the hormone that helps labor progress)
- Increased levels of endorphins (your natural epidural)
- Slower breathing
- Adequate blood and oxygen supply to the uterus and your baby
- Uterine contractions are effective (the muscles are working together)
- Shorter labor and reduced pain - feelings of wellbeing

Why is it that most animals seem to give birth relatively easily and without a lot of drama? A cat will seek a private warm environment to birth her kittens and will even purr while giving birth. Even in the wild, an animal that senses a predator will stop labor and won't give birth until it feels safe. What do they know that we don't? They certainly haven't taken any prenatal classes and, as far as I know, there hasn't been a "feline" edition of *What to Expect*. I always enjoy having families from a farming background or dog breeders in my workshops because they get to see first-hand how the animals in their care can usually labor easily and quietly when they are undisturbed. Sometimes the farmer's enthusiasm about how easy natural birth is for other animals can be incredibly annoying to their partner – so there's always some fun banter to be had. When a veterinarian joins the class the too understand that most of their involvement is to just observe discretely from a distance, being careful not to interrupt the process.

Next time you visit the zoo, ask the keepers about their protocol for when one of their rare mammals is about to give birth. In most cases, they observe by camera or from a distance so as not to disturb the mother.

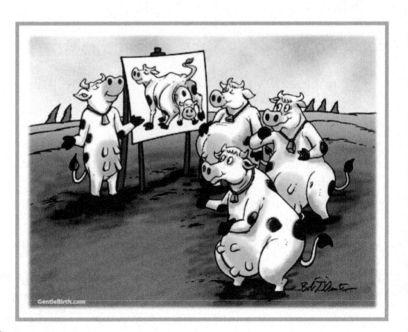

SENSATIONS IN LABOR

Like many moms using GentleBirth for the first time, you probably believe you have a really low pain threshold - you might think that you just don't "do" pain very well (brain bully alert)!

Many women do experience birth as painful, others experience it as quite manageable, and some women even find it relatively painless, but their experience of pain in other areas of their lives rarely translates into how they cope during the birth of their baby. Why assume you won't be able to cope? When was the last time you heard a woman talk about giving birth as an enjoyable and manageable experience? (I hear it a lot!). And, if you did, what would your reaction be? Probably that the men in white coats should be along soon to take her away. Mothers who have comfortable births are dismissed as lucky, liars, or delusional.

Women openly planning an unmedicated birth are smirked at with knowing glances that say, "Just you wait…. you'll be begging for an epidural" and

are warned that "There are no medals for going without." No doubt you've heard about these amazing medals and root canals without medication. Would you have an epidural because of strong period pain? That's how many GentleBirth moms experience most of their labor. A common misconception for homebirth moms is that the pain of labor is necessary and even empowering. Yes, pain is a great communicator that directs your body movements but, in a normal, healthy labor, extreme distress and pain (as seen on so many TV shows and described in so much detail on every pregnancy online discussion) do not have to be present.

PRIMING

Every day we are subjected to millions of messages and as we absorb them they have a profound subconscious influence on how we behave. Advertising works, even when we're not consciously aware of it. Being exposed to certain words can influence how old or how young we feel. In one study, participants walked slower after being exposed to words associated with the elderly. There is also an opposite effect for youthful words: participants walked an average of 10% faster leaving the experiment. A few words can have a direct effect on how we think and behave. You are unconsciously primed to feel like a patient the minute you walk through the doors of a hospital.

In GentleBirth we use a much softer language: we talk about contractions or surges – some moms like the term 'uterine waves'. The word contraction creates an image in the mind of contracting, constricting, and getting smaller but lots of moms still prefer to use that term especially with care providers. I really think they should rename them "expansions" because the body is opening up, not closing up.

GentleBirth moms focus on releasing and relaxing. Waters don't "break," they release; and mothers experience a birth show instead of a bloody show.

The majority of GentleBirth moms describe their sensations during active labor (generally the most intense stage) as uncomfortable. Doula and childbirth educator Desiree Andrew says, "It is true that naturally occurring labor can feel larger and greater than the woman birthing. This is not so, as she creates from within the very hormones that increase the strength, power, and frequency of her work of labor. That is the good news: It is from her, for her, by her. It is the might of creation moving through you."

PAIN ONLY EXISTS IN THE BRAIN

"What your brain is doing in labor is just as important as what your body and baby are doing"
−Tracy Donegan−

In her book, Dynamic Positions in Birth, Margaret Jowitt describes the uterus as a '3-dimensional trampoline' and the surges 'fold' baby back into the middle for the easiest birth.

Think about those trampolines with springy netting on the side (to stop you falling out); those elastic walls force you back into the center of the trampoline.

The muscles of the uterus like all muscles in the body were designed to work comfortably. Saying that pain only exists in the brain is not about dismissing or trivializing women's very real experiences of pain in labor. But as the research in pain science evolves we're discovering that we can use the brain to reduce all kinds of pain including labor pain. Your brain is responding to information received by the senses, your previous experiences, emotional state, culture, focus and support will influence how much pain you feel in a healthy normal labor. Basically the brain makes an educated guess about and how much danger it believes you're in and that will either increase pain or reduce it. It might surprise you to learn there are no pain receptors in the uterus – but there are nerves that are activated by different kinds of stimulus 'mechanical' (pressure/stretching), thermal (heat/cold) and chemicals (prostaglandins). Toward the end of pregnancy, your body down-regulates almost all of the nerves in the uterus as your body ramps up oxytocin receptors.

These nerves do remain in the cervix but few remain in the uterus itself. This information often has every mom in my class puzzled – because if there are few to none of these nerves in the uterus why do so many women experience labor in such a painful way?

Biology dictates that fear and anxiety increase adrenaline production in the body, which then creates a physical reaction by activating the fight/flight response. In preparation for defending itself, the body starts redirecting blood flow away from our organs to the limbs. The uterus is not a defensive organ and, just like the heart, cannot work effectively, comfortably, and efficiently when blood is restricted and the muscles spasm.

Each cell in your body has receptors - these are like locks and keys. The cells are the locks and the keys are your hormones. Hormones 'dock' into these cells like a spacecraft docking with the space station.

If oxytocin gets to the cells first, it's like putting the key into the ignition of your car: It starts the engine and gets things moving, causing your uterus to surge effectively. If the adrenaline key gets to the cell first, it blocks the ignition so the car is much harder to start and keep running well.

When there is adrenaline present, your body's built-in epidural (endorphins) can't co-exist and it slows the release of oxytocin needed to help labor progress. It's almost like driving with one foot on the brake and one foot on the accelerator. Even women who plan on unmedicated births prepare themselves to "embrace" the pain as if it is inevitable. Midwife Jan Tritten describes it well.... "The battle is in the mind - at birth, we are unblessed with a thinking mind."

As adults, the mind is the biggest obstacle to a positive pregnancy and birth. We listen to others, watch "Baby Story" on television, hear of cesarean rates and the ease of epidurals, and completely lose our ability to do the task for which our bodies were supernaturally designed.

I sometimes hear from midwives and childbirth educators who have never witnessed a calm, focused GentleBirth that pain exists so that mothers know they are about to give birth and they can get to a safe place - so that their babies don't just drop out on the supermarket floor...

GentleBirth mothers experience sensations but, in most cases, it is not perceived as unbearable, excruciating pain. These mothers are very tuned in to what's going on in their body as they are more mindfully present to the sensations.

Another popular belief is that mothers who birth through painful labors are somehow transformed into confident, strong, empowered mothers. But what of the mothers who birth without discomfort? Are they less empowered, less confident mothers? Is it pain in birth that brings about this transformation in the mother or is it the experience of being fully present in mind and body, birthing instinctively and confidently that brings about new growth?

Extreme pain does not always exist in a healthy spontaneous birth but, when there is pain, it's trying to communicate something to us. When you are calm and focused you can hear what your body is telling you. Pain is communicating that there is something not quite right that needs to be attended to. Sometimes it's as simple as adopting a different position to make yourself more comfortable or shifting your pelvis around your baby as your baby rotates and spirals within.

Neuroscientists suggest that pain in labor exists for the following reasons:

- It provides feedback to drive changes (changing position, moving).
- A protective sign that there 'may' be danger.

- Drives help seeking behaviors (most moms will seek out the support of their partner and midwife/OB.

PAIN IS AN OUTPUT OF THE BRAIN – NOT THE UTERUS.

It's an opinion of the brain, a best guess. That output is based on context, on perception, and we all perceive things differently including pain. Back to that Facebook debate about THE dress? A study by Schlaffke et al. reported that individuals who saw the dress as white and gold showed increased activity certain parts of the brain associated with more sophisticated thinking (I'll go with that analysis!). Your brain is basically trying to decide is this something we need to be worried about? If the brain concludes that yes this is life threatening your pain will increase and if it concludes that it's something exciting the pain will decrease. So how you think about labor pain will change how you experience labor.

"There is power that comes to women when they give birth. They don't ask for it, it simply invades them. Accumulates like clouds on the horizon and passes through, carrying the child with it."
–Sheryl Feldman–

TWO APPROACHES TO PAIN IN LABOR

There are two very different approaches to pain in labor. There's the medical model that sees pain as associated with something going wrong, damage to tissues and should be eliminated immediately. The medical model doesn't recognize that emotions, beliefs or culture have any impact on how we experience pain. Then there's the 'working with pain' model that suggests pain is a normal part of labor and is productive, positive pain and women have the resources to cope with it when they feel safe and well supported. This model recognizes that emotions, thoughts and labor support will impact our experiences of labor pain. Of course we can't talk about pain without talking about suffering. I agree 100% with the medical model here – in this day and age given the resources we have available in the modern world no woman should experience suffering in labor and yet it happens more than we'd like to admit. Pain can exist without suffering – when you are working hard during labor but you're focused and coping you're not suffering. Suffering happens when you feel overwhelmed, out of control and don't have the resources and/or support to cope. That's why building your labor toolkit in pregnancy is so important.

▌DIMS & SIMS

It has nothing to do with your Saturday night take out but an innovative approach to understanding pain. In their 'Explaining Pain' work Neuroscientist Lorimar Mosely and David Butler have come up with a creative approach to how the brain assesses signals from the body. He calls them DIMS and SIMS. A DIM is something the brain sees as a 'danger in me message' and a SIM is a 'safety in me message'. In labor is the brain producing more DIMS or SIMS?

DIMS and SIMS can be things you see or hear in labor, things happening to your body, your beliefs, how safe you feel.

Moseley and Butler propose that you'll experience more pain (DIMS) when your brain comes to the conclusion that there is credible evidence of DANGER (birth being very dangerous) than SIMS (birth being normal and the sensations are associated with something positive. What is it about stepping on Lego that sends the brain into a frenzy of DIMs. Not even the biggest and best neuroscientists have figured that one out.

Go to your GentleBirth workbook now and take the DIM/SIM exercise.

When predicting which moms would need medication in labor researchers found that above all, pain catastrophizing was found to be the strongest predictor of requests for pain relief.

WHAT DOES LABOR PAIN MEAN TO YOU - THE STUFF OF NIGHTMARES OR A CHALLENGE?

At this point you should be starting to see which model of pain resonates most with you – the working with pain model or the medical model of pain. As your pregnancy progresses you may find you're drawn to one more than the other. If you're using the GentleBirth App regularly you may find you're feeling more positive about unmedicated birth or feeling more confident about getting further in labor without meds – but as always see how you feel on the day. You might just surprise yourself!

I like to have moms imagine how they imagine themselves in labor? When those thoughts pass your mind do you see yourself as focused, working hard but coping or feeling distressed, distracted and distraught? This might be a good time to complete the Mental Rehearsal exercise in your workbook.

FEAR OF LABOR AND BIRTH IS A LEARNED BEHAVIOR

Your brain is already trained (wired) for fear in labor (it's a learned behavior) – you weren't born with the fear of birth. You learned it over and over again. The brain evolved for survival, not happiness, so we have inherited some behaviors from thousands of years ago such as the negativity bias which means your brain is always on the lookout for threats. This old 'legacy brain' is like the factory settings on your phone but thankfully, due to the extra plasticity in pregnancy, we can do some DIY brain remodeling during pregnancy. It's like body sculpting but for your brain. You're bulking up in some areas (parts of the brain associated with decision making, positive mood, emotion regulation, and slimming down other areas. At GentleBirth, we're all body positive but in this circumstance having a skinny amygdala is a goal worth working toward. The less blood flow this part of your brain gets the smaller it gets so you're literally shrinking your fear in a physical way.

A healthy expectant mom living in the developed world is rarely in physical danger yet her amygdala (that smoke alarm) cannot tell the difference between a piece of toast that's burnt or the house is on fire...it starts shrieking anyway. The amygdala can't tell the difference between an angry bear chasing you in labor and stressful thoughts about labor and birth, financial worries etc. Your body reacts as if you're being chased by a real bear. In pregnancy, this panic, stress, and the recurring hormonal cascade of adrenaline impact your unborn baby too (chronic stress is a major contributor to preterm and low weight babies in the US).

LEARNING TO 'SWITCH'

Let's talk about two important networks in the brain that can make or break your pregnancy, birth and parenting experiences. You have a 'default mode' and 'focused mode'. Default Mode Network is what we're in about half of the day your mind is wandering and worrying. The focused mode is called the 'Task Positive Mode' - that's the network of the brain that gets activated when you are focused on what you're doing.

Some examples of default mode would be when you read the same page of a book and can't remember what you just read. You're worried about going to the dentist next week. You're in a meeting and thinking about the big proposal you have to finish up by the end of the day and your colleague called in sick. You're on your phone scrolling through Facebook watching a movie at home and you've no idea what's going on in the movie.

Focused mode is when you are paying attention to your experience right now. When you're washing the dishes, you're washing the dishes – not thinking about that credit card bill. When you're in labor, you're paying attention to your breathing or you're focused on movement - you're not thinking about how long more it's going to take. Professional athletes spend a lot of time in focused mode.

At the GentleBirth workshop, you and your partner will learn more about the 'Switch' technique and other strategies to instantly move you out of default mode and into focused mode. The more often you use each network, the bigger it grows and the research shows that, the more time we spend in default mode, the greater the risk of anxiety and depression. It's a case of use it or lose it.

> "Giving birth should be your greatest achievement,
> not your greatest fear."
> –Jane Weideman–

PAIN AND THE BRAIN

Pain exists only in the brain and the brain decides what the sensation means – something it perceives as good or bad (non-life-threatening or life-threatening). How you've trained your brain will influence whether your brain thinks the sensations of labor are to be welcomed or avoided. We know this is true because of the ongoing research on phantom limb pain experienced by amputees. Brain scientists have even written case studies on women's experiences of menstrual pain - after a hysterectomy.

Our experience of pain is determined by several factors:

The fear of labor is a learned behavior - you learned it from family, friends, and TV shows. Pain depends on how much danger your brain "thinks" you are in, rather than how much pain actually exists. Based on what you've learned about birth over the years, your brain will react in an appropriate way.

Consider this scenario: At 41 weeks, a first time mom starts to experience tightenings and sensations she has never experienced before. The stretch receptors (there are very few pain receptors in the uterus at full term) in the uterus sends a signal to the spinal column like a relay race. It passes the signal up through the brain to the thalamus, which acts like a relay station or a skilled air traffic controller who decides where the signal goes next. On receipt of the signal, the thalamus asks the pain committee how serious this signal is - is it something we need to be worried about? For the majority of expectant moms, the rest of the brain responds immediately with "YES!! YES!! THIS IS REALLY, REALLY BAD, birth is all about blood and tearing and pooping and being out of control and in horrible pain. It's just like that TV show we saw." So your mental meerkat sends an excitatory message back down to the uterus saying, "Keep it up, keep it up!! This is something awful and we need to make this mom take notice!" Just like the children's story about Chicken Little, your brain thinks the sky is falling.

GentleBirth moms usually have a different experience, especially when labor starts on its own.

At 41 weeks, a GentleBirth first-time mom starts to experience tightenings and sensations she has never experienced before. The uterus sends the same signal to the spinal column, which like a relay race passes the signal up to the brain. On receipt of the signal at the thalamus, the brain asks the pain committee how serious this signal is.... is it something we need to be worried

about? The rest of the brain responds quite differently, saying "Cool - this means the baby is coming and we're so excited! This is something really good." Mental meerkat relaxes and says "Tell those guys down below to CHILL OUT" - and sends an inhibitory signal back to the uterus because these sensations are not something we need to be worried about. (Adapted from the work of Professor Lorimer Moseley).

> "The exact amount or type of pain depends on many things. One way to understand this is to consider that once a danger message arrives at the brain, it has to answer a very important question: "How dangerous is this really?" In order to respond, the brain draws on every piece of credible information – previous exposure, cultural influences, knowledge, other sensory cues – the list is endless." –Dr. Lorimer Moseley

Expectations or beliefs that a procedure will be painful amplifies or turns up the perception of that sensation (it's the brain trying to predict the future again). Most GentleBirth moms experience the sensations of birth as uncomfortable and intense (and powerful) and most first-time moms who prefer to have an unmedicated birth in the hospital do so successfully.

YOUR EMOTIONAL STATE – EXCITED OR TERRIFIED?

Imagine you have just received the news that you have lost your job. Panicked and in shock, you trip over a box in the hall and twist your ankle - imagine the pain you might feel. Now imagine you have just found out you won the lottery and, in your excitement, you jumped up and down and twisted your ankle. Which experience do you think would be the most painful?

A GentleBirth mom recounted a story of how she tripped and broke her ankle a week before her wedding. Immediately after the fall, mom attempted to stand but she was restrained by her partner, who insisted that she stay sitting. Mom felt she had a slight sprain - nothing serious - how could it be, she was getting married in a week? As she looked down, she realized her foot was hanging off her leg at a very unusual angle, but she still insisted everyone was over-reacting. She was embarrassed by the trip to the hospital in the ambulance and spent the time apologizing to the paramedics for wasting their time and wondering how she would finish up the final wedding preparations with a sprained ankle. The ER doctor informed mom that she had a tib/fib fracture (both bones of her lower leg were broken) and she would need immediate surgery. As the realization of her injury sank in and what this would mean for her wedding, mom began to feel excruciating pain - pain that had not existed moments earlier. Mom was so focused on her wedding next week that the brain couldn't process the pain signal.

The emotional state you are in determines how much pain you experience (or if you even feel any). Depending on your emotional state, your brain will interpret the information differently and with less or more intensity. The calmer and more focused you are during the birth process, the less intense the sensations can be and the more manageable everything is.

How Much Attention You Give the Sensations (or in GB speak – WTF – Where's the Focus).

Brain imaging studies show that when we focus on painful sensations the area of the brain associated with pain processing receives more blood flow and the sensations are felt more intensely. However, when participants are instructed to focus on music rather than the painful stimulus, the intensity of the pain is significantly reduced.

This is why it is so important to use your brain training during the birth process if you find you need some help staying focused.

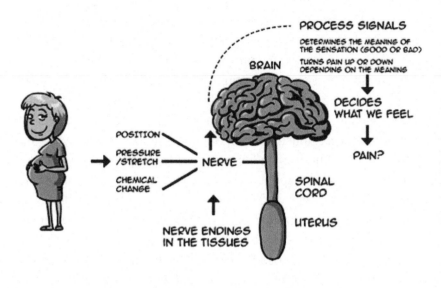

"People always say that pregnant women have a glow. And I say it's because you're sweating to death."
–Jessica Simpson–

I CAN DO ANYTHING FOR A MINUTE

Sensations are subjective, I do not presume to tell you what your labor will feel like. Every woman experiences labor differently. GentleBirth does not promise pain-free birth; if you follow the program and do the daily training, you will certainly feel calmer, confident, and more in control which often translates into a more manageable experience but more importantly you'll have all the tools you need for a positive birth. GentleBirth techniques are tools intended to help you work with your body and stay connected to your baby with or without medication. The epidural is a wonderful tool - but it's just one of many - and you have lots of tools in your GentleBirth labor toolkit.

Doula Jennifer Cook de Rosa brilliantly describes how manageable birth can be. The thought of labor pain is scary. The fear alone can be enough to choose medication (in the hospital parking lot if available!) without considering how much you can manage and how long it will last. Once you are in established labor, you will experience sensations that come with regularity.

From the time a surge/uterine wave begins until the time the next sensation begins will determine "how far apart" the surges are. Let's look at this more closely.

Surges are coming every three minutes and lasting for about one minute. This means that, in one hour, you will experience surges for 20 minutes, and will be resting for 40 minutes.

A surge has an "up" (like the cycling uphill imagery earlier) when it begins; a tightening. Then it has a "peak" where you feel its intensity, and then it goes "down," which is relaxing. About half of the surge is "up" and about the other half is "down" with only a second or two at the peak. Only half (the first half) of your surge will involve the "discomfort." The other half is relaxing.

Since you can estimate 20 minutes of the hour is spent surging, only half of that time is spent on going "up." In other words, 10 minutes out of every hour!!

Make your mantra "I can do anything for one minute." The "up" of a surge will almost always be less than one minute except maybe during the final minutes before birth.

By taking your surges one at a time and spending the remaining part of your labor relaxing, you will find that labor can be manageable. Be sure to relax completely between surges... let your body go totally loose and limp so you can conserve your energy, listen to your brain training or favorite music, and breathe nice deep rhythmic breaths.

ACTIVE LABOR

Surges usually coming about five minutes apart, lasting 45 seconds (23 seconds "up");

55 minutes of rest, pressure felt for five minutes per hour (you can handle that!)

Surges coming three minutes apart lasting 60 seconds (30 seconds "up"); 50 minutes of rest, discomfort felt for 10 minutes per hour (10 minutes per hour...that's all).

THE HOME STRETCH

Surges coming two minutes apart, lasting 90 seconds (45 seconds "up") 37 minutes of rest, intense sensations felt for **23 minutes per hour** and, at this point, you're on the home stretch and will be meeting your baby very soon.

"So the question remains. Is childbirth painful? Yes. It can be, along with a thousand amazing sensations for which we have yet to find adequate language. Every birth is different, and every woman's experience and telling of her story will be unique."
–Marcie Macari–

CREATIVE MIND GAMES

Hypnosis - It's Not What You Think.

Hypnosis can help replace negative attitudes and emotions by decreasing anxiety, tension, and panic before, during, and after birth. Let me help you understand the logic behind hypnosis, your subconscious mind, and your wonderful imagination. It is not pro- or anti-religion.

The only way to change the 'programs' you already have (anxiety of birth/ parenting) is to record over them. That's where GentleBirth comes in. You are recording over the old programs with new programs and "upgrading" your mental software from fear to confidence, both consciously with your mindfulness practice and CBT and unconsciously with hypnosis. (BTW hypnosis is so much easier than meditation).

The more you practice, the quicker the new programming takes effect and you don't have to think about it - it's automatic.

Think about when you first learned to drive. Do you remember consciously thinking of everything you had to do and what an effort it was? After a while, you got more comfortable and it got easier; a few weeks later, you were driving without having to think too hard. Everything you'd been practicing so often became a subconscious activity - no thinking required! As the GentleBirth programming starts to take effect (within a week or so), you find your attitude changing and your excitement growing. When you begin to feel those first sensations of labor, all of your practice pays off as you remain calm, confident, and in control.

WHAT DOES HYPNOSIS FEEL LIKE?

In two words - very normal.

Have you ever found yourself daydreaming? When you're daydreaming or focused on that exciting new book you're reading or the latest episode of your favorite TV show, even though you are perfectly aware of what's going on around you, you're in what's called a "light" trance. With GentleBirth, you are cocooned in confidence and outside distractions just fade away into the distance. We go into hypnotic states several times during the day and do not even know it's hypnosis. Watching TV is the most common form of hypnosis and marketing companies are well aware of this.

The feeling of daydreaming is exactly what it's like when you are practicing self-hypnosis for birth. It's like watching an interesting movie one that you're fully engrossed in and time passes quickly and pleasantly. You experience an overall feeling of calmness throughout your entire body. At all times you are totally aware of what's going on around you. You are in complete control and you can communicate clearly and effectively with your birth partner and - when the time comes for you to have your baby - with the medical team supporting you. As a technique for complete body and mind relaxation, which is really very important in childbirth, hypnosis is a great tool to have in your labor toolkit.

WHAT'S SO IMPORTANT ABOUT YOUR SUBCONSCIOUS MIND?

You are aware of your conscious thinking but not aware of your subconscious thinking, which makes up 90% of your mind but it is running the show behind the scenes - just like the Wizard in "The Wizard of Oz." The subconscious is the part of the mind that we're working with for your GentleBirth.

Your subconscious mind regulates all involuntary bodily functions, including your heart rate, breathing, blood pressure, hormone production and release (prostaglandins, endorphins, oxytocin, and adrenaline), digestion, and the elimination system. The subconscious mind is self-protecting. It has to be, because the subconscious is the home of your ability to breathe, digest food, and pump your heart... It will protect you from real or IMAGINED dangers. Think of how your heart races and you sweat when you're having a nightmare - your mind is telling your body it's real, even though you KNOW that monster isn't real (but your mental meerkat is sounding the alarm anyway).

HOW THE MIND WORKS

Your conscious mind is the part of your brain where you make all of your decisions - like what to have for dinner, or where to go on vacation. It's also the home of your short-term memory - your current phone number, your current address.

We think it's the conscious mind that's in control when, in reality, it's just a small part. The larger part of the mind that controls all of your bodily processes is run by the subconscious mind.

Your subconscious mind is also where your emotions (fear or confidence) and your feelings are stored.

It's also where your permanent memory is stored, so everything that you have ever been told about childbirth over the years and the images and emotions you have formed because of these influences are stored within your subconscious mind. If you've heard nothing but scary birth stories, that's what your subconscious believes - and that is your reality.

The brain and nervous system respond only to mental images. It doesn't matter if the image is imagined or real. While you're watching "Grey's Anatomy" or "One Born Every Minute," your mind thinks it's real. Another way to think of it is imagining your subconscious being like your computer hard drive. You have had various programs in your mind since you were a child; some are good and some are not so good. Hypnosis can be like doing a virus scan on your computer; it finds any corrupt programs or programs you don't need anymore (negative beliefs about birth) and updates the old programs.

The subconscious mind is very lazy and won't accept new "beliefs" without constant repetition (that's why following your daily brain training is essential). In hypnosis, we do all the work with the subconscious mind once we get past the "bouncers." The skills you are learning in the GentleBirth program should be practiced every day for the best results.

Can you commit to 20-30 minutes of practice every day for the biggest event of your life (keep in mind it's 30 minutes cozy on the couch or in bed drifting into the most relaxed state you've ever been in)?

The subconscious mind is like a 2-year-old - it believes EVERYTHING, whether it's real or imagined. It doesn't judge, rationalize or try to make sense of it. If you are constantly watching scary birth shows on TV or reading scary birth stories you are reinforcing to your subconscious mind that long traumatic, distressing labors is a fact and that is your reality. Just reading scary birth stories changes your physiology. That's why visualizing your calm, confident GentleBirth is so important.

*Note this is not a birth preparation version of 'The Secret' – thinking about an amazing birth does not guarantee it will happen but you'll definitely enjoy your pregnancy a lot more and you and your baby will be exposed to a lot less of those stress hormones. Birth is unpredictable - if things did change for you on the way would you feel like you wasted all those weeks feeling uplifted, calm and confident? Of course not.

THE SUBCONSCIOUS MIND – WHERE THE MAGIC HAPPENS

Between the conscious and subconscious mind are filtering mechanisms, or protectors. These are the "bouncers" or gatekeepers that protect your subconscious mind. They are very selective about what they let into the subconscious mind and they are also very lazy: They only like to let in suggestions that are like the ones already inside, such as the belief that birth is an ordeal. The only way we can replace the negative birth beliefs is to get past the bouncers, which is what we do in hypnosis. So we wait until they go on a break (hypnosis) and we slip past and make the changes easily. We remove fear and replace it with confidence. Once in hypnosis, the changes happen easily. The conscious mind makes no judgments about the new beliefs, it just runs the virus scan on your mind, updating it with new and improved programs that work for your benefit. Combined with mindful practice and actively challenging the birth bullies, you're shifting your perspective on birth completely.

WHAT DOES THIS MEAN FOR BIRTH?

Many women experience labor as an ordeal - in part because we expect it to be like that. If the mind repeatedly expects something negative to happen, then it becomes a self-fulfilling prophecy. So, if you expect an excruciating ordeal of pain, then that's usually what you get. If you expect it to be manageable and have prepared well physically as well as mentally, you build up a positive mental expectancy of childbirth and change the negative programs in your "computer" (subconscious mind) and through hypnosis you upgrade your subconscious thoughts to new confident feelings and imagery about birth.

Using your imagination is like a birth "dress rehearsal" of the mind and the big secret to having a positive birth is to imagine or picture this happening over and over again. This is part of the conditioning process.

In a famous scientific experiment from the 1950s, a baby was conditioned to be afraid of white objects simply by exposing the baby to a loud noise and a white object at the same time. It only took seven exposures for this newborn to "learn" to be afraid of white objects (a coat, a dog, etc.). How many times have you been exposed to scary birth stories episodes on "Grey's Anatomy" or "One Born Every Minute," etc.? Most of us learned at a young age that birth was something to be very afraid of.

Mental rehearsal is similar to methods employed by the greatest athletes in the world. By using self-hypnosis techniques throughout your pregnancy, you can change the old beliefs you have built up over time by visualizing how you want your birth to be.

So when the time comes to give birth for real, your body and mind are so familiar with the images of calm, relaxed childbirth that your physical body reacts to these images automatically by completely relaxing all your muscles and producing your own natural anesthesia (endorphins).

During birth, it's much easier for you to remain relaxed, calm, and in control, because this is what you've retrained your body and mind to do.

▌CAN I BE HYPNOTIZED?

You may be reading this and thinking that you're too smart, analytical or Type A to use hypnosis, but most people can be hypnotized if they are willing participants and have a curious easy-going attitude to it; but, as with any skill, some of us are better students than others.

Most people can be hypnotized. There are two main criteria for success with hypnosis: - intelligence (you need to have an IQ above 70), and the need to address any fears about hypnosis. You obviously have no lack of intelligence and have an IQ above 70 or you wouldn't have chosen the GentleBirth program. Fears are usually addressed through understanding how the mind works. If you have any questions or need any clarification, please feel free to contact me.

Another common misconception is that you are unconscious or asleep during your GentleBirth. In hypnosis, you are, in fact, more alert than during your normal state of awareness you hear the suggestions in your training you decide if you like them and accept them if you do.

You cannot get stuck in hypnosis; if you were listening to your training and the doorbell rang, you'd either ignore it or go answer it.

Your brain training sessions are simply guiding you into a state of self-hypnosis - which you'll easily learn how to do yourself.

You have to WANT the suggestion to work ... the word TRY will block the suggestion, it means you have doubt. As Yoda says, "You must do or not do - there is no try."

During pregnancy, you are probably very conscious of what you put in your body. Now it's time to become more conscious of what you put in your mind. Consider GentleBirth to be a mental and emotional fitness program - and, just as with any fitness program, the more you put into it, the more you will get out of it.

Each day you have a choice to choose to feel positive or not. It's always a choice. In preparation for your GentleBirth, we encourage you to choose to focus on better-feeling thoughts. Just lean in the direction of a better- feeling thought. This is not "Pollyanna" thinking but "intelligent optimism," which has documented health benefits for you and your baby.

USING POWER THOUGHTS AND AFFIRMATIONS

Imagination is everything.
It is the preview of life's coming attractions.
−Albert Einstein−

What is an affirmation? An affirmation is basically anything you tell yourself on a regular basis, both positive and negative, and, the more often we say it to ourselves, the quicker it becomes a belief. Imagine if you have a habit of saying to yourself that you're not very good at something. How often do you find yourself saying something like "I'm always late," "I'm so disorganized," etc.? We tend to focus on the negatives. Every word, action or behavior is an affirmation because our thoughts and imagination create our reality. A positive affirmation is a strong, positive statement that something is already so. It is positive, personal to you, and in the present tense. The more often you say it with the appropriate emotion, the sooner it becomes a new belief.

HOW DO AFFIRMATIONS WORK?

Write a list of things you DO WANT for this birth and create positive suggestions for yourself. It's very easy to come up with the list of things you DON'T want but what DO you want? What's important to you about this birth?

> Some suggestions for your birth affirmations;
>
> I am calm confident and in control in all circumstances.
>
> My baby is the perfect size for my body.
>
> My labor is powerful – I am strong.
>
> I release all fears and trust my body and my instincts.
>
> I tune in to my body and tune out distractions. My baby is healthy.
>
> I am prepared for whatever path my birth shall take.

Positive affirmations are used to program your subconscious mind. The continuous process of replacing the negative thoughts with positive affirmations is essential.

It takes practice but it gets easier and it will positively affect every aspect of your life. It might feel a little strange in the beginning, but keep it up! You control your thoughts or they control you and you have approximately 50,000 thoughts a day (most of them are repetitive). By ignoring or challenging the negative thoughts, we are refusing them energy. This is like not watering a plant. The plant eventually dies from lack of water (attention and focus), like those brain circuits. By continually changing the negative thought and affirming the positive thought, we can form a new habit in the subconscious mind within a few weeks. The old habit of thought dies because we are not giving it energy, that old neural pathway in the brain withers and dies as the new GentleBirth neural circuits grow bigger and bigger with the new activity. By being aware of our negative thoughts, we have the power to transform them into powerful tools of change. Affirmations are far more effective when you can connect a positive emotion with these power thoughts. Simply repeating a sentence day in and day out has limited impact. The brain responds to emotion, - and will take those new affirmations on board if there is an emotional component. Think of a time in your life when you felt very in control, imagine that scene... where you were... bring up those feelings as strongly as you can. Where do you feel it in your body? As that emotion builds, repeat your affirmation to create that link in the brain so the brain can associate that affirmation with those feelings automatically. The subconscious mind is filled with all sorts of old "programs" about birth that our parents and other people programmed into us when we were young. So long as it's there, all this old programming from early childhood is controlling your present life.

You control your mind or it controls you. Professional athletes have known this for years and use visualization and positive self-talk regularly. A study in the U.S. showed that athletes who use positive self-talk are more likely to make the Olympic team than those who don't. Of course, we shouldn't expect to be the 'thought' police and have to monitor every thought we have. The easiest way to know if your thoughts are positive or negative is by how you feel. Your feelings are like a GPS or an emotional satellite navigation system in your car. When you are thinking about something positive, you feel good, and when you're thinking about something negative, you feel bad. It's that easy!

> Is what I'm focused on now making me more excited or more anxious about my baby's birth?

*"The whole point of woman-centered birth is the
knowledge that a woman is the birth power source.
She may need, and deserve, help,
but in essence, she always had, currently has,
and will have the power."*
–Heather McCue–

I CAN DO THIS - EXERCISE

As you intentionally bring up memories of achievement in your life, you are creating powerful connections in the brain. One of the biggest predictors of achieving a goal in any area of your life is a previous track record of success in any area. In other words, we don't have to have faced the same challenge before to feel confident that we can deal with what we're facing now. Resilience comes with that feeling of knowing that you have been successful in the past and can be successful again in the future. Don't focus on what you did but how you felt when you realized that you had done it. It can be anything at all - something you feel good about when you think of it - that feeling of "I did it." Go on and let yourself take some time for some personal bragging - it's all in the name of science and your positive birth. As you bring up these memories of a time when you coped really well with some event in your life, you are intentionally calming down any mental meerkat activity.

If your birth partner is supportive, encourage that partner to come up with some birth affirmations for himself/herself for his role as birth partner, new parent, etc.

Some suggestions for birth partner affirmations:

- I remain calm, confident and focused as I support my partner through each phase of labor.

- I am confident in our plans for our birth and in my ability to convey them to our caregivers.
- I know my partner is capable of giving birth in a healthy, safe and peaceful manner.
- I know that I will respond to her needs and requests with our baby's best interest in mind.

BIRTH STORY

They Told Me I Was Too Calm to Be in Labor

I didn't listen to the App during labor because I was told in the hospital I wasn't in labor. I went to the hospital at 2 pm with broken waters, I was told I would be induced the following day if I didn't go into labor. I thought I was in labor with the surges I was having and the nurse told me they were just like strong menstrual cramps, I wouldn't be so calm and be able to talk.....

During the 'menstrual cramps,' as they called them, I would repeat in my head "I can do anything for a minute and I know how to birth and my baby knows," and did reiki on myself. The nurse told my fiancé to go home at 1am to rest before my induction, it was going to be a long day. I never had a vaginal examination to check my dilation. The baby's heart rate was checked when I arrived at hospital and was high, they checked it again when I went to the ward around 5pm and not sure when the next one was, think about 9pm, the time got lost in my head after 7pm. After my fiancé left, the pressure from the surges got more intense and I felt nauseous. I walked to the nurse's station and asked for a sick bag. I felt as if I need the toilet and to push but was sharing a ward with five other women that needed the bathroom. I rang for the nurse and a different midwife came. I was leaning at the window and said can I get a Motrin. She asked me what my last dilation was. Told her I was never examined. My midwife came and asked what the problem was. I told her I need to push and she asked would I like a shower or to sit on the birth ball!!

The other midwife said, "I think this baby is doing super things and fast." Then, with the next surge, I squatted and grunted. The midwife went running out of the ward, yelling "Get my girl a room!" She came back and told me I better ring my husband. He said he got the call at 2am. The other midwife had got a wheelchair. I said I had to walk; I couldn't sit. So I walked to the delivery room, leaned over the bed; then they said get on the bed, put on the monitor and the baby was in distress and I was 10cm. An OB came and asked had I just come in like this and called for vacuum and forceps. She introduced herself and said there was going to be a lot of people coming into the room. There was people shouting "Push!" and I had no contractions so I didn't, I was in my own world, focused on my own surges and pushing when they heightened. Then I heard head was out, shoulders out, body, and I was looking into blues eyes screaming at me. Lucky my fiancé and I live five minutes drive that he made it and cut the cord. Baby Adam was born at 2:26am, 26 minutes after I rang my fiancé. Adam had a scratch on his head and cord bloods checked, and doctor looked over him, he had been 15 minutes in distress that they knew of. But he scored 9 on APGAR. Then the questions started, the OB asked what my method was, I had been doing hypnobirthing or some method because she could see it in me. What was my diet, the bloods were some of the best she has ever seen. What exercise I did because only for the distress I had an episiotomy but I wouldn't have torn. She said I was built to give birth and that all my efforts with diet, exercise, acupuncture, and GentleBirth stood to me that night. Only for my efforts and ability to focu,s keep calm and do what I had to she predicted there would have been a different outcome. Adam stayed with me and my fiancé and didn't require neonatal. All my work had paid off. She told all the staff to congratulate me. And told my fiancé I did an amazing job and she knows my baby would be thanking me. Everyone I've told my story to knows someone that is pregnant and scared of labor and I have recommended going to your website. And they are amazed I walked in and out of the delivery room, in my ward of four, I was the only natural birth and my baby was so alert compared to the other babies there. He never left my side and I could walk around with him, I never felt any pain and was on a high for days. It never seemed as if I had just had a baby. Next time in bold type I will have on top of my birth plan 'I HAVE DONE GENTLEBIRTH, LISTEN TO ME WHEN I SAY I'M IN LABOR!'

- "I had my second gentle birth nearly four weeks ago. I was in the prenatal ward already when I went into labor and I keep remembering this interaction with the midwife who had just started her rounds. I walked down the room and asked her if she'd come check on me, she replied, yes hon, I'll get to everyone don't worry. I said no I think things are happening, can you check me now, please. So she puts me on the trace and can see the contractions so she examines me. The look on her face as she tells me I was 5cm. I bet she never had someone at 5cm walk up to her before! Thanks to gentle birth for keeping me so calm and helping me to trust my body and my baby"

- "I walked into the labor ward, went to the midwife and told her I'm in labor. She laughed at me and said, 'You wouldn't be able to tell me you were in labor if it was true'. My husband got annoyed and asked if they can check, she said okay, she put a monitor on, saw how frequently I was getting contractions ... eventually started believing me... decided to check more, I was 6cm dilated and had my first baby boy two hours later!"

THE LAWS OF THE MIND

Every Thought Causes a Physical Reaction

Take a moment or two and think of a really embarrassing experience from your past and notice how your body reacts just to the memory of the experience.

Your heart rate may increase; your face might even become flushed. Your thoughts affect all of the functions of your body. Constant worrying creates excess acid in the stomach, which often leads to digestive issues. When you are angry or upset, you stimulate your adrenal glands and the increased adrenaline in the bloodstream causes body changes, including reduced immune function and increased tension. Anxiety and fear increase your pulse rate and breathing and they direct blood to your arms and legs (fight or flight) and shut down digestion. Thoughts of your favorite foods start your tummy rumbling and your mouth begins to water. Sexual thoughts ...you get the picture. These are just examples of the mind-body connection.

You Get What You Expect (that fortune telling brain again).

The subconscious mind responds only to mental images (images of scary births or GentleBirths). It does not matter if the image is real or not. The mental image formed when you were younger becomes the blueprint and the subconscious mind uses every means at its disposal to carry out the plan. Worrying is the repeated programming of an image you do not want.

The subconscious (not knowing the difference between a real or imagined image) acts to fulfill the imagined situation and "The things I feared most have happened." With the above law in mind, the statement takes on new meaning.

YOUR IMAGINATION IS MORE POWERFUL THAN KNOWLEDGE

The mind works best with imagery. Images are the language of the subconscious mind. Those images will always override what you think. Reason is easily overruled by your own imagination. You've probably spent a lot of time imagining what childbirth will be like; were any of those images positive ones?

Any thoughts that are accompanied by a strong emotion e.g. fear, generally can't be changed through the use of reason. (Even though we know factually that birth is quite safe in the Western world, it's still frightening for so many).

This is one of the reasons why GentleBirth works so well. You are reducing anxiety and creating a positive expectation that birth can be empowering and positive, no matter what happens on the day.

ONLY ONE IDEA OR EMOTION CAN BE EXPERIENCED AT A TIME

This does not mean more than one idea or feeling cannot be remembered or held in your memory. You can choose to focus on negative thoughts or be aware of your thoughts and change them when you realize you're having a negative thought. You can think of your partner lovingly in one moment and then remember a time that they upset you and the feeling may not be so "loving," but you can't experience both emotions simultaneously. This can be helpful to the STOP technique, too. Try to feel appreciation in that moment and you'll change the way you react and the chemical cascade that started when the driver cut you off. You get to choose to continue the negative thinking or change the thought and emotion associated with that event. You take charge of your emotional spotlight. The brain simply doesn't have the bandwidth to process competing signals.

"GentleBirth was fantastic. I felt totally in control and calm and ready. The hospital completely adhered to my birth plan and the midwife did as asked and didn't offer me anything other than support and her hand to squeeze! It was very quick and was painful but my body did what it was supposed to do and when baby emerged I was totally pain-free walking around, in and out of shower and baby on boob in no time!"

HYPNOSIS TRAINING

Before we get started, there are a few things to remind you of. The most important thing is that hypnosis is a state of mind that requires your full participation. It's not a nice story that you're listening to in the App or if you're using the exercises at the back of the book. When I ask you to imagine or visualize something, really imagine it. Do not drive while following your brain training unless they specifically state they are safe to use while driving. Choose different times of day to listen to the program (not just at 10 pm at night when you're in your favorite PJs in clean sheets). We don't want you creating a conditioned response that you can ONLY get that relaxed when you're in those PJs late at night in the fresh sheets. Find a place where you can get comfortable. Let yourself focus on the program. Let go of any other thoughts of the day.

Make yourself a priority for this time. I want you to be completely engrossed in my words, to begin with, as you would be in an interesting movie. You'll find that your mind wanders and that's fine (it's so much easier than meditation). You may find your hands get tingly or heavy. Many moms experience time distortion 30 minutes seems to feel like 10 minutes. When you have been practicing for at least two weeks, it's fine to use your hypnosis brain training while doing something repetitive, such as ironing or even going out walking, but do commit to spending that time each day on you. Some moms report feeling emotional - this is a good sign - the new programs are taking hold but still bumping up against the old, long-held beliefs. You may find your eyes fluttering; some moms feel warmer.

You may also notice that your breathing slows down to a nice comfortable rate. Many moms say they feel better during their practice time than they ever have.

You'll find you sleep more deeply than ever before.

Whatever the signs, these are all indicators that you are responding to hypnosis really well. You will find yourself feeling more confident after your daily session. If you're wondering if hypnosis is real or not, let's look at that now: Have you ever been driving and missed the turn because you were daydreaming? Have you ever been so engrossed in a movie that you screamed when a scary part happened or cried during a sad part? (Who hasn't cried during the movie "E.T."?)

As mentioned earlier, you should think of GentleBirth as a mental and emotional fitness program, but this is a fitness program where you see the results immediately. They are skills that can last a lifetime, as long as you choose to use them. Most moms start to feel more confident and relaxed within a few days of starting their brain training.

Take a really easy-going attitude to your practice but make a commitment to following it daily.

If you don't experience what you think you should experience, just relax and go with the flow. Just listen to the words, dim the lights loosen your clothing, take your shoes off, get comfortable. This is YOUR time. Allow yourself to be 100% committed to preparing for your baby's birth. As with any fitness program, the more you put into this, the more you'll get out of it and hypnosis training is so much easier than mindfulness, which demands ongoing continued focus.

Enjoy your hypnosis training - you're already on your way to feeling calmer, more confident, and more in control in all areas of your life. If you haven't started already, this is the perfect time. All you have to do to is open, play, smile, repeat.

HIGH-TECH BIRTH

Virtual Reality

Technology is changing our world in ways nobody could have imagined. 10 years on no one could have predicted how reliant we would become on our little palm-sized devices called smartphones that have become such a huge part of our lives. Apps followed and now there's an App for everything. If you've been to one of my workshops, I've been talking about VR, distraction, and pain perception for years (Snow World and the penguin snowball game). I met Hunter Hoffman, the creator of Snow World, at a recent Stanford VR conference. Hunter pioneered the use of VR for acute pain in children with severe burns with incredible results.

Angry Birds Anesthesia - Will Fruit Ninja Replace Fentanyl?

A few years ago, I witnessed a very quick and seemingly comfortable birth with mom using only a Playstation DS for pain relief. Mom was completely engrossed in her game and as her brain can only process a limited number of signals – pain signals were significantly reduced. We already know that smartphone Apps can train your brain for less anxiety – but with the advances of VR, pain reduction in labor is now a reality.

Virtual Reality Birth

For some women, VR may be extremely effective for labor and it looks like we may have more answers in the near future from ongoing research. In 2016, Erin Martucci relaxed on a virtual tropical beach as she labored in a New York hospital supported by her OB with no medication. One hospital in Arizona recently started a study for pain management in labor and a study comparing perineal repair with analgesic, and VR was very positive with moms feeling significantly less pain. A 2017 study in Wisconsin proved to be very successful for first time moms planning an unmedicated birth.

With all of this impressive new research, it makes sense that trials are beginning for the use of VR for labor pain and anxiety (before or during labor). The brain has limited 'bandwidth' and can only focus on one stimulus at a time, so combining relaxing imagery with positive suggestions and sounds of nature can significantly reduce pain. We know that anxiety and fear in pregnancy increase pain in labor (and even complications) - so why not use technology to change that as part of your birth preparation. Some psychologists have been using VR for several years to help patients overcome phobias and extreme anxiety - birth preparation could be much more enjoyable when experiencing it by a beautiful lake at sunset or while sitting on a tropical beach.

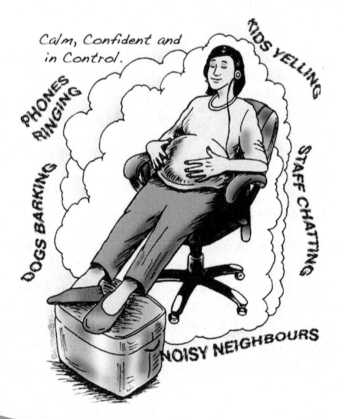

BREATHING TECHNIQUES

You may be surprised to learn that there don't have to be any complicated breathing techniques for childbirth. That's right, no counting, just slow focused breathing. When you are in a relaxed state, you don't need any techniques. Full abdominal belly breathing is our normal state when we arrive in the world but stress changes it quickly. Think of a time when you ran up a flight of stairs - at what point did you think to yourself, "I now need to redirect my blood flow and change my breathing pattern to oxygenate my muscles" or did all of this happen automatically? Your very clever body just adjusted your rate of respiration to the work of your body. When there is no excessive adrenaline in the first stage of the birth process and you are calm and focused, your body will do the same. Only when you lose focus or get stressed do we need to introduce any kind of breathing techniques that you'll be learning in your brain training. They are simply another tool in your labor toolkit to use if needed. Having a wobbly moment – slow down the breathing. Be sure your partner knows this too.

Imagine you have a nose on your bump to remind yourself to breathe all the way down to your baby. Here are some simple reminders for slow relaxed breathing during your practice and during your baby's birth.

SIMPLE BREATHING MEDITATION

I know I just said we won't bother with counting when it comes to breathing but this is a mindful breathing practice so the counting can help you be more aware of how often your mind wanders. Today each time you get stuck at a red light or feel the need for a bathroom break take 3 deep breaths. Notice the sensation of the air entering your nose or the feeling of your belly expanding as you breathe in and the sensations of the air leaving your body. Just let your body breathe you. Try to stay with it gently. Like a puppy on a leash, your mind will want to bounce around so sometimes counting your breaths can be helpful in this exercise. Start at 1 with the in breath and 2 for the out breath...and count to 10 slowly. As you become aware of your puppy mind chasing other thoughts simply start over again with 1. The most important aspect of this exercise is not to get to 10 perfectly every time but to be gentle with yourself and non-judgmental when you find your puppy mind has gone off chasing cars (thoughts). As you practice this exercise you are training your mind to stay focused on one thing at a time and be present on purpose. This is a great exercise to use after your baby is born too.

The average adult takes between 12 and 20 breaths while resting, depending on your emotional state and fitness level. As you breathe in, your heart rate speeds up and, as you breathe out, your heart slows down. Simply by lengthening your outbreath, you can optimize that relaxation response. Time yourself, whatever your current rate of respiration, make a commitment to yourself to practice slow comfortable breathing over the next few weeks and try to bring that number down. Some moms find it helpful to focus on a word, e.g., "Relax." Focus on the 'Re" when breathing in and "Laaaaaax" when exhaling or try counting (you'll find that in the App).

THE JUST-IN-FROM-WORK BREATH

If like most GentleBirth moms, you're holding down a full-time job (at home or outside the home) and growing a baby, you'll already have lots of practice with this breathing technique. It's that long outbreath that you take as you finally put your feet up after a long day.

Slow Breathing

Slow breathing, just like it says, is slow easy breathing as you move into a stronger rhythm of birth.

Birth Breathing

The eye-popping, purple-faced pushing often seen on TV is no longer recommended. Long periods of holding the breath restrict oxygen to your baby and exhausts mothers. The uterus is a smooth muscle; this means that you have no conscious control over it, unlike the muscles of your arms and legs that you can flex at will. It's similar to other areas of smooth muscle in your body, such as the inside of your stomach and intestines. Smooth muscle is also found in your blood vessels. All smooth muscles have one important function: They squeeze your blood, waste, food and yes, even your baby along its path.

You didn't have to consciously move your sandwich down into your stomach and through your intestines; it's all involuntary. As your cervix thins and opens, the opposite is happening to the top of your uterus (fundus): The top of the uterus grows thicker.

Think of your uterus as a tube of toothpaste that has to be rolled up behind the toothpaste to get the last bit out - or an image I love is to imagine the uterus like a big icing bag and it's smoothly pushing the pink icing out through the funnel. Even the walls of the birth path act differently during a surge compared to the relaxed state between surges. When relaxed between surges, the interior walls of the birth path look like folds of pink tissue; they look corrugated and, during a surge, these walls stretch out to look like a smooth pink slippery slide. Will the corrugated or smooth pathway make it easier for your baby to move closer to being in your arms? When we think of the birth process and hear of labors lasting days, it almost seems like your baby is arriving from deepest darkest Peru! In fact, the distance your baby has to travel is about the length of your middle finger.

When your body opens to full dilation, your uterus gently moves down behind your baby and starts to involuntarily nudge your baby down the short birth path. As this is happening, you begin to feel a new sensation of pressure in your back passage, as if you need to go to the bathroom. Our instincts are to immediately hold everything and panic because God forbid that we are going to poop in labor! It means that your baby is very close to being born. (As a midwife I can tell you when I see poop - I'm happy!) It's gone in a flash and not something to worry about at all. Baby is on the way.

Birth breathing means working with your own urges and only nudging your baby down when it feels right for you letting your body do the work. Some nurses still coach moms to hold their breath and "push into your bum." We are the only mammal that does this and we're now realizing that it is not beneficial to moms or babies. Have you ever seen a dog barking at another dog having puppies to hold their breath and push into their bums!

"Women's bodies have near-perfect knowledge of childbirth; it's when their brains get involved that things can go wrong."
–Peggy Vincent–

BODY

YOUR PELVIC FLOOR

Looking after your pelvic floor now, before you give birth, can save you weeks, months, and even years of problems, such as incontinence (leaking urine when you sneeze or cough). It can also mean the difference between getting your "groove" back in the bedroom in a few weeks OR a few months. The pelvic floor is made up of a sling-like band of muscles at the base of the pelvis, attached to the area of the outlet. These surround the anus, vagina, and urethra in a double figure-eight pattern.

These muscles support all the woman's pelvic and abdominal contents, and the baby passes through them during birth.

BENEFITS OF HAVING WELL-TONED PELVIC FLOOR MUSCLES

- Helps your baby descend during the second stage of labor.
- Prevents stress incontinence.
- Can increase sexual satisfaction.
- Can prevent prolapse of pelvic organs.
- Helps the perineum to heal faster after birth.

YOUR PELVIC FLOOR

We have all heard of the "pelvic floor," but what exactly is it? The pelvic floor refers to the muscles of your pelvis, whereas the pelvic girdle refers to the bones. When we put our hands on our hips, we are actually putting them on the top of the pelvis, the iliac crests. The word pelvis comes from the Latin for "basin" and it can be helpful to visualize the bones of the pelvis as the "walls" and the pelvic floor muscles as the base.

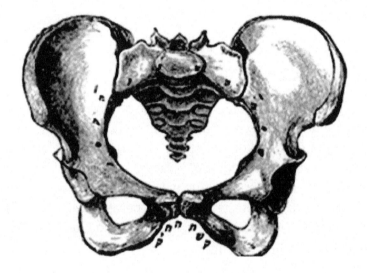

There are three layers of pelvic floor muscles, running from the tailbone (the coccyx) to the pubic bones at the front.

There are three openings or sphincters in the female pelvic floor, one each for the bladder (the urethra), the uterus (the vagina) and the bowel/rectum (the anus).

The pelvic floor muscles have a number of functions, including controlling the opening and closing of these sphincters. They also support your pelvic organs (your bladder, uterus, and bowels) and help maintain strength and stability in your lower back, along with your lower abdominal muscles. The pelvic floor and deep abdominal muscles are commonly referred to as your "core" muscles.

During pregnancy, the pelvic floor muscles have to work hard to support the weight of your growing baby, to maintain control over your bladder and bowel so you don't leak, and also to help stabilize your lower back and pelvic girdle - the bony structures of your pelvic region. The pelvic floor muscles also have a role to play in sexual function - they have to relax enough to allow penetration into the vagina and then contract during orgasm. As your baby moves down and out through the vagina, it's important that you know how to find and relax these muscles, because they need to be flexible enough to stretch to allow baby out.

There can be a lot of conflicting advice over whether or not to do strengthening exercises for the pelvic floor - some women do need to strengthen the PF muscles, but most women just need to learn how to coordinate them - as with any muscles, if we just practice tightening and strengthening, this can lead to inflexibility and stiffness - not ideal for birth!

BENEFITS OF PELVIC FLOOR COORDINATION

- Improves control and prevents leaking from the bladder and/or anus during pregnancy and after delivery
- May help reduce tearing, especially when combined with perineal massage
- Improves sexual enjoyment during and after pregnancy
- Reduces back pain during and after pregnancy
- Easier bowel movements
- Faster recovery after birth

HOW TO DO KEGELS CORRECTLY

Research has shown that the best way to contract your PF muscles is to close the openings and then lift up and in. It is not a good idea to stop and start mid-stream when you are urinating, as this can lead to bladder problems and infections.

Most of your PF muscles are actually located toward the back of your pelvis, so it can be easier to start by imagining you are trying to stop yourself from passing gas.

Always start by relaxing! Take a deep breath in and, as you exhale, relax all the muscles around your pelvic floor.

Take another breath in and, as you exhale, try to close the openings of your pelvic floor, then imagine you are lifting up and in - think of an escalator moving from your tailbone toward your pubic bone at the front of your pelvis.

Hold the muscles up and in as you breathe.

Then (and this is the most important part) let the muscles relax again completely.

WHAT IF I STILL HAVE PROBLEMS FINDING THE MUSCLES?

Try some of the following exercises and see if any of them help you get a proper contraction:

Try sitting close to the edge of a hard kitchen chair and imagine lifting your pelvic floor off the chair surface.

Imagine lifting a marble into your vagina (just imagine!)

Sitting in a chair, place your fist or a rolled-up towel between your knees. Lean forward a little and take a breath in and out to relax. On your next exhale, squeeze your knees together and see if you can carry that tightening all the way up to your pelvic floor. Don't hold your breath as you do this! Don't work too hard when you are doing your PF exercises! Putting too much effort into a pelvic floor muscle contraction can actually lead to the wrong kind of contraction, which is called a "Valsalva" maneuver. A Valsalva maneuver is a bearing down technique similar to having a bowel movement when you are constipated (if you are doing your Kegels correctly, there should be a lifting up, not a bearing down). If you are having difficulty performing a Kegel, put only 50% effort into each contraction, go slowly and gently, and use your breath. Your PF muscles automatically contract a little with every exhale, so exhale with the contraction when you are doing your exercises. You are much more likely to achieve the correct type of contraction this way. And, as always, don't forget to keep breathing through the exercises and always relax your pelvic floor afterward.

HOW OFTEN SHOULD I DO MY PF EXERCISES?

There is no evidence to suggest that there is a "magic number" of repetitions. Some guidelines suggest doing 10 slow contractions (where you contract the pelvic floor for up to 10 seconds) and 10 fast contractions (where you squeeze and quickly release, squeeze and quickly release, etc.) anywhere from three to eight times a day.

The key seems to be doing your exercises (and not forgetting to actively relax the muscles) little and often throughout the day. Some women find it easier to remember to do them after each meal, others when they hear an ad break on the radio or TV or when they hear a phone ring. Try and find a "trigger" that happens regularly throughout your day, such as flushing the toilet or washing your hands.

TOILETING TECHNIQUE

Practicing coordinating using your PF muscles when you are having a bowel movement is an excellent practice for birth! During labor and birth, the ideal is to be able to use the breath and abdominal muscles to help baby down and out when you feel the urge (but never by holding your breath to push) but to keep the PF muscles relaxed when you are doing this. Every bowel movement can be a mini-rehearsal for birth.

You should never hold your breath to push during a bowel movement - even if you are constipated.

When you are having a bowel movement, it's ideal to have a small stool or step that you can rest your feet on, so that your hips are slightly and comfortably higher than your hips.

Lean forward so your elbows are resting on your knees.

Push out your belly, as if you are trying to make your waist bigger.

Take a breath in and, as you exhale, relax and soften around your anus.

Keep breathing deeply in through your nose and out slowly through your mouth as if you are smelling the flowers and blowing out the candles.

The digestive tract starts at the mouth and ends at the anal opening, so be sure to relax both ends of the tube. Place your tongue on the roof of your mouth with your teeth separated. This helps relax your mouth and will help to relax the anus at the same time

As you feel the feces moving down and out, keep breathing and give a grunt (or try using other sounds, such as ahhhh, shhhhh, ohhhh, or grrrrrrr).

BIRTH STORY

First-Time Mom's Wonderful Experience

When I found out I was pregnant with my first child, I did what I do with everything and I researched as much as I could about pregnancy and labor. I do a lot of exercise and sport and I wanted to keep fit and make the experience as positive as possible. I came across the GentleBirth program while reading on the Internet and decided this was for me. I considered going to the workshop but I was a bit skeptical how well it would work on me, so I decided to buy the tracks and book and go through it myself. I read the book (twice!) and any bits I thought my husband should know about I read them out to him (he is not the 'sit down and read a book type'!). To be honest, the whole concept was so interesting it became a constant topic of conversation for us and it tied in a lot with our approach to training for sports endurance events, which was great. I tried to read some of the GentleBirth birth stories too but, at the time (over two years ago now), I couldn't really find any first-time mothers that had used the program. The majority of people seemed to have had a bad experience with their first labor and had used the GentleBirth program to help with their second. As the time got closer, I listened to the tracks more and more and I found it fantastic - really relaxing. I was so positive about the whole pregnancy and how I felt and I really think the tracks helped with that. My due date passed but myself and my husband had focused on the due date + 2 weeks date as the endpoint, so we didn't really think about it passing. Three days later, I woke up feeling a bit crampy but it was so mild I didn't even know if it was anything. After a couple of hours, though, it seemed as if the cramps were coming at regular intervals, so I started to time them and could see there was a pattern. It looked as if it was starting but I knew it could take a long time to get going so I just hung out at home relaxing. By lunchtime, the pains had stopped and for a couple of hours nothing was happening but I still couldn't face eating food or going anywhere so I stayed put and, sure enough, they started back up. By the evening time, I was sitting in the baby's room in the dark on the rocking chair chilling - my husband came home from work and checked to see if I needed anything but I was fine. The contractions were coming about 5 minutes apart at this stage but totally manageable. My husband was canceling his evening arrangements but I felt so fine that I sent him out and told him I'd let him know if I needed him. I continued timing them and relaxing and by 10pm I thought it was time to head to the hospital. One thing I did have a slight fear of was being trapped in the car in a lot of pain but the car journey was lovely! I don't even remember having any contractions during it - we were just chatting away as we drove. The hospital was completely empty when we arrived and so quiet. I was admitted and checked but only 3 cm, so I was brought up to the delivery suite and introduced to the midwife, who read through my birth plan with my husband and went out to change to another midwife because she had done a hypnobirthing course! I was in the Rotunda and I know there are different experiences everywhere but I found them amazing and totally open-minded to what I wanted. They left myself and my husband alone for hours, kept it all dimly lit and didn't offer me any pain relief, which was all part of my plan. For the next few hours, I labored away. The contractions were really close together and I found I was too uncomfortable to sit or lie down and rest and didn't have time for a breather in between but I kept focused and kept thinking I was getting closer to the end. A few hours in, I asked my husband to get the midwife and see if there was any progress being made. At that point, I was getting really tired and I needed something to keep me going. I decided to take some of the gas and air and that was amazing! It gave me a great break and slowed my breathing right down, which is exactly what I needed. Still laboring away but no real progress so, in the end, we asked the midwife was there anything she could do and she offered to break my waters. I went through all the pros and cons and decided I would go ahead with it and the minute she did it we were straight into the final stage. An hour or so later at 6am, our little boy arrived. Perfectly healthy and I was completely fine too. I took a shower, had some tea and toast, and walked to the post-labor ward - I felt great. It was tough at times for sure and looking back I would have done some things differently (like eat and get some rest earlier in the day as well as stick on my GentleBirth tracks earlier) but overall it went exactly as I wanted it and was such a great experience for all of us.

Part II

Two years later, we welcomed another little baby into the world. Of course, I used GentleBirth again and found it fantastic. When my due date arrived, the doctors started offering me sweeps this time and it totally threw me as it wasn't something I had even considered. But I explained to them that I wanted no intervention unless it was totally necessary and asked them if there was enough fluid and a good heartbeat. Once I knew our baby was healthy, I declined the sweep and didn't even let them examine me, as I have heard of women being examined and by accident or because they thought they were being helpful the doctor has done a sweep anyway. I asked them how long they would let me go past my due date and they said 10 days but if there were no issues, they would consider two weeks. So I kept going with my plan of no intervention and hoped I would go myself. To be honest, I did have a wobble at one point. Was I being crazy holding out to go myself, was I putting the baby in danger for the natural birth, was I taking unnecessary risks? So I mentioned it to my husband who gave me a talk down. We had discussed everything about the GentleBirth plan and doing things as naturally as possible, provided there was no risk involved, so he knew exactly what I wanted and was completely on board with it. He was the perfect person to talk to about it and, once he had finished, I felt so much better about sticking to our guns on this. But it wasn't easy at times when the doctors looked a bit surprised that I didn't want any interventions. Having said that, the midwives we spoke to were all incredibly supportive and all agreed that our approach was the best plan A to have and anything after that could be dealt with then. The morning after myself and my husband's chat I went into labor - fantastic! I woke up again with contractions and, once we had our son sorted in crèche, I closed our bedroom door, turned the lights out, got into bed and put on GentleBirth. Straight away, the contractions calmed down and got further apart. It was amazing. I listened to the tracks for hours and after a while I started to visualize hard rippling sand on a beach with a wave of water flowing over it for each contraction. Sounds crazy but it really worked to make each one totally manageable. I switched to listening to a song playlist I had prepared to take a break from the tracks and even started getting a bit emotional at the songs - it really was a euphoric experience - it's the only way I can describe it. At about 3:30pm, I felt the need to get up and walk around. Things were ramping up a bit so I said to my husband that maybe we should head into the hospital. He had left me to it all day and just brought me food when I texted him downstairs (I wasn't making that mistake again)! So I was all fuelled up and ready to go. Into the car and I just listened to the tracks all the way in, completely calm. When we got to the hospital it was 4:30pm. I was admitted and examined and was 6 cm, which was amazing. I was chatting away to the nurse and she was asking how long I was in labor the last time. We said 'a few hours' and she was saying that she didn't think it would take that long this time and she'd get us up to the delivery suite straight away. We were only in the door of the delivery suite doing the introductions and I asked for the gas and air. The minute I hopped up on the bed I could feel huge pressure. I sucked on the gas and air and I must have taken so much of it in I blacked out for a minute. When I came around, I had to actually ask my husband what was happening and he was like 'the baby's head is almost out!' One more push and he was out in the world - we had been in the delivery suite for 6 minutes!! It was phenomenal. I think we were all in shock, but again he was perfectly healthy and I was fine - no stitches again and had a shower and walked to the post-labor ward. It really was the perfect experience.

To be honest, all along I've been more afraid of being tied to a drip, of having to labor in a labor ward with other people after being induced and needing surgery/having stitches than I ever was of labor itself and so the GentleBirth program was the perfect program for me and my boys. Even with my first labor, I felt it really helped with my enjoyment of my pregnancy and staying completely relaxed throughout it. It can be hard to explain to people how amazing labor can be when you do it like this and, of course, if there had been any need for intervention I would have taken it but, as I said, as a plan A to me it's the only option. I recovered so quickly from both deliveries and there were no complications for either of my boys. It was more difficult, I felt, for my first pregnancy as you are trying to relax into something and you don't quite know what that is! But it is definitely possible and by the second time around it was just perfect from start to finish. I am so thankful to GentleBirth for both of these experiences.

FIT BITS (AKA PERINEAL MASSAGE)

Where Is the Perineum?

There's not many women who look forward to this conversation but if you can get past the cringy feeling taking this part of your birth preparation seriously can pay off. The perineum is the skin around the entrance of the vagina between the anus and vagina. During childbirth, the perineum stretches and unfolds gently to allow the baby's head to be born...the slower the better. Mention perineal massage to most moms and almost all of them will squirm in their seats. But a few minutes of perineal massage in those last few weeks of pregnancy can make the difference between being able to squirm in your seat and having to sit on a cushion for three weeks.... and an intact perineum makes sex more likely much sooner (maybe you've sworn off sex at this point in your pregnancy and that's not much of a motivator so don't do it for your sex life – do it for your recovery and pelvic floor health).

What Is a Perineal Massage?

Perineal massage is stretching the skin to improve the elasticity of the tissues and to get you familiar with the sensation of stretching you feel when your baby's head is being born. It's particularly important if you don't have a very active lifestyle. It may not sound appealing but can help you avoid a tear or episiotomy, especially for a first baby.

Perineal massage should not be done if you have a vaginal infection, a herpes sore, or any other vaginal condition that may be spread or worsened by the massage.

The massage should be started sometime in the last trimester, at least 3-4 weeks before the due date, 2-4 times per week is enough.

Not everyone is comfortable with this practice, so discontinue if discomfort persists.

Some women find that they like to incorporate the massage into lovemaking but do not like to do it themselves, while others find that they like to do it themselves so that they are in control. The important thing is to do what works for you.

TRY THIS TECHNIQUE

Scrub the hands, trim the thumbnails, and sit in a warm comfortable area. Relax with your legs apart in a semi-sitting position. To become familiar with the perineal area, use a mirror for the first few massages. Use a pure vegetable oil or a water-soluble lubricant (not a petroleum-based oil) on the fingers and thumbs and around the perineum. Use olive oil or coconut oil or an organic product, because KY jelly has parabens (hormone disruptors) and glycol in it - up to 20% of women have glycol sensitivity and there is some evidence to link glycol use in lubricants to vulvodynia.

Vegetable oils are easily absorbed by the tissues, enhancing the suppleness achieved by the massage.

Spread enough oil over the perineum to allow the fingers to glide easily. The perineum is the area behind and outside the vagina, toward the anus. It is not necessary to go near or touch the anus.

Avoid touching the anus followed by the vagina because the bacteria that normally live in the digestive tract can cause an infection in the vagina (and UTIs).

Using the index fingers or thumbs, insert them into the vagina up to the second knuckle, or as close to that as is comfortable. Press them against the back wall of the vagina and slowly sweep them away from each other up the vaginal wall as they are pulled outward gently. The movement is a sort of "U" shape. This movement should be repeated for several minutes. This is similar to what you may feel as the baby's head presses down before it starts to emerge from the birth canal.

Next, rub the perineum between the thumb and forefinger, one finger inside the vagina and one finger outside. You can use one hand or two. Then place two fingers just inside the vagina, only to the first knuckle, and gently stretch the perineum outward. Massage more with the thumb and forefinger if the tissue feels tight. Remember to consciously relax the muscles, using slow breathing if the sensation feels a little too intense.

As the tissue gradually relaxes and stretches after several sessions, apply more outward pressure on the perineum to cause a stretching sensation. This is the sensation many women feel as the baby's head stretches the perineum during crowning. This is the time to use birth breathing until the stretching sensation eases. Some women may suffer a tear at this point in a birth because they don't anticipate the stretching sensation and they jump, reflexively tightening their perineal area. You should relax into the sensation and know that, when you feel it in labor, it means your baby will soon be here.

Being too vigorous could cause bruising or swelling in these sensitive tissues. During the massage, avoid pressure on the urethra as this could induce irritation or infection.

Kegel exercises can be added to the routine to help get the feel for the pelvic muscles. Do this ritual once or twice a week beginning around Week 36 of pregnancy.

As your bump grows bigger and it's harder to reach, you can stand up; put your foot up on a low stool or step and reach around to your perineal area from the back.

Visualize warm oil being poured on your perineum... all of the muscles relaxing completely with the warmth of the oil and your baby slipping gently into the world and into your hands.

(Thanks to physiotherapist Michelle Lyons for her collaboration. For more information, visit Michelle's blog at michellelyons.wordpress. com or speak to Michelle in the App.)

WHOLE, HEALTHY, AND INTACT - PROTECTING YOUR PELVIC FLOOR IN LABOR

Perineal trauma in modern birth has become so commonplace that moms almost expect that they will need some 'help' in this last very important part of birth. Hollywood has us convinced that all that purple-faced pushing is normal. The second stage of labor becomes a frantic race to get the baby out as quickly as possible - suggesting to women that their own body is a danger to their baby. Your body has grown your baby from two cells to a perfect baby ... knowing exactly where each fingernail should be placed ... where your baby's tiny ears should be placed ... down to the perfect number of hair follicles on your baby's head ... with no conscious input from you ... no 'fetus growing' classes ... just the intelligence and wisdom of your body. For most women your body also knows how to finish the process.

Over the years I've worked with a few moms who have had serious ongoing complications of incontinence after a traumatic birth - in many cases, it involved an assisted delivery with forceps or vacuum. As perineal injury becomes 'normalized,' we are losing sight of how physically and psychologically debilitating a damaged pelvic floor can be in day-to-day life and in a woman's relationships with her partner.

Sadly some moms feel it was partly their fault because they couldn't 'push' properly or were too uptight and couldn't 'let go'. So let me start off by stating that your body works. Your body knew exactly what to do and in most cases so did your baby. You weren't too 'uptight' or had issues with letting go. Your body did not fail you - routine birth practices most certainly did. Even the most skilled yoga moms and the most laid-back relaxed hypnomoms are faced with the most challenging intervention in current obstetrics - not the forceps - but the clock. What most moms don't realize is that they are on a time limit from the moment they are 'diagnosed' to be in labor until the placenta is delivered - the clock is ticking. There is no evidence to support these arbitrary time limits.

Here's a typical scenario that plays out in delivery every day. Mom is managing well - baby is healthy and coping well with labor. Mom has two hourly VEs (vaginal exams) to ensure she is dilating with the hospital's guideline of 1cm per hour (there is no evidence to support 2-hour VEs). Around 7cm (sometimes even at 10cm) mom's labor slows down as her body rests and her baby rotates into the optimal position mom is deemed to have inefficient uterine action and is prescribed IV Pitocin and her waters are broken (there is no evidence to support doing this).

Mom is now on continuous electronic fetal monitoring due to the administration of IV Pitocin. Mom is finding it more difficult to cope (and may feel she needs an epidural) with the chemically driven contractions that give her and her baby little or no rest between. Baby finds it harder to recover from the intense, longer chemically driven contractions and is now showing late decels on the CTG.

Mom is now 10cm and baby is showing signs of distress due to the longer intense contractions of the IV medication. Additional staff enter the room and mom is instructed to lie on her back and pull her knees up to her chest as two nurses instruct her to hold her breath and push into her bum (whether she has any urge to push or not).

Sometimes staff will tell mom to 'get angry with her baby'. Prolonged breath holding further restricts oxygen to her baby, which again shows baby in distress and a decision is made for an assisted delivery. An episiotomy is performed and vacuum applied - vacuum fails and forceps applied. Baby is born limp and has low APGAR due to hypoxia (lack of oxygen). Mom is in a state of shock but thankful that her baby was 'saved.' Mom's notes read - 'FTP' - failure to progress - and reluctantly accepts that this was her fault - she's just one of those women who need a lot of help to get the baby out...

Nobody told mom that holding her breath for long periods of time could put her baby at risk. Nobody told her that 'purple pushing' could damage not only her baby, but her bladder, her pelvic floor, and her perineum. In fact, the prenatal classes encouraged it and other women told her to 'listen to your nurse - she'll show you how to push'.

Current evidence and international best practice would suggest that this was a case of 'failure to wait' rather than failure to progress. In my experience, there are several factors that increase the risk of perineal/ pelvic floor damage.

Arbitrary time limits (time limits mean more assisted deliveries).

Coached pushing.

Overuse of episiotomies. Evidence does not support the use of routine episiotomies.

Overuse of epidurals and underuse of hydrotherapy (water immersion is associated with lower perineal damage).

There are a number of studies comparing coached vs. spontaneous pushing. In 2003, the WHO recommended removing coached pushing from practice. Research from 1957 describes the damage to the muscles of the vagina and support ligaments after coached pushing, so the new research is reaffirming what we already knew to be the case - that 'purple pushing' is harmful to women and their babies and the more moms can educate themselves about local practices the better. I often hear moms saying not to focus on the birth as it's 'just one day'.....but that's not the case for those women who are living

with incontinence for the rest of their lives. My recommendations are the same to all women whether they have had previous trauma to the pelvic floor or are first-time moms.

It's helpful to understand how the 2nd stage of the birth process actually works.

IT'S A REFLEX

Just like that knee reflex your doctor checks and you involuntarily kick, when your baby's head triggers Ferguson's reflex, your body automatically starts to nudge your baby down. The top of the uterus gets thicker and thicker and moves down around your baby - like a tube of toothpaste. Think of how our body works when you feel sick and vomit. Your body throws up ... so in labor it's like your body is throwing 'down'. You'd never say, "Oh, I had food poisoning last night and was pushing up vomit all night" ... you'd say you were throwing up and I'm fairly sure you never took 'effective vomiting' lessons. It's the same with the 2nd stage of labor ... your body does all the work for you. You can't NOT go with it.

It's an irresistible urge that you can't ignore. Think of how the bowel works - pushing when you don't have the urge to push is like someone instructing you now to go and have a bowel movement immediately when you don't feel the need to go! Think of a time when you really really needed to go ... did you need someone to coach you? Did you need to do anything else other than sit down and relax? Whether you sit on the toilet and push for America or bring a book (partners are usually skilled in this area), the poop still comes out!!! When you think of it, how did humans get born for the thousands of years before nurses and doctors came on the scene? Who is coaching the cows and sheep in the fields or the women who have accidental homebirths or give birth in the car? Mother-led pushing is protective for your baby. When you hold your breath for sustained periods of time the oxygen to your baby is turned off.

TIPS FOR FIT BITS IN LABOR

Practice perineal massage in the 3rd trimester (especially if this is your first vaginal birth).

Information is not power ... applied information is power. Write your birth preferences down and discuss prenatally; e.g., "I prefer not to have coached pushing but will push with my own urges."

Ask for more time if you and baby are well.

Allow your birth partner advocate for you in labor if a staff member starts instructing you to hold your breath.

Choose an upright birth position even with an epidural (yes, this is possible - discuss this with your caregiver).

Ask for more time if you and baby are well.

Focus on slow comfortable breathing - let your body do the work.

If you have an epidural, request additional time for 'passive descent' also known as laboring down, especially if you and baby are well.

Ask for more time if you and baby are well (getting the picture?)

Labor in water if possible even if water birth is not an option or something you're not comfortable with.

Consider a homebirth, birth center, or private hospital midwife scheme or if possible, choose an obstetrician/midwife with a low rate of episiotomies and assisted deliveries to stack the odds in your favor.

GentleBirth Mom

"No matter what sort of labor you have or what type of birth you want, this program cannot fail to help. I wasn't particularly concerned about having a drug-free birth, but I did want to be confident and relaxed throughout my pregnancy and labor no matter what happened. I definitely achieved this by listening to the GentleBirth program. I never imagined I would be so relaxed that my husband would be taking photos of me in labor about to go to hospital at 3am! A fantastic program".

TURN ON YOUR BIRTH HORMONES
BRAIN HACKING FOR BIRTH

Hypnosis and meditation slow brain wave patterns bringing about a meditative state that calms the sympathetic nervous system (turns off your fight-flight response).

Positive expectations of a calm GentleBirth - the more painful you expect the experience to be, the more pain is experienced.

Slow diaphragmatic breathing turns off adrenaline (short shallow breathing means less movement of the torso for mammals under threat so they are visible to predators).

Laboring in warm water shortens labor considerably by hacking into your natural oxytocin which shortens labor.

Aromatherapy lavender and rose essential oils contain chemicals known to have a sedative action on the brain. Jasmine/clary sage can encourage more efficient surges during birth if needed.

Humor releases endorphins.

Blueblocker glasses may help increase melatonin production (and will definitely be a talking point if you go for the Bono rockstar look in labor).

Massage releases endorphins and oxytocin.

Familiar surroundings lead to feeling safe (oxytocin release).

Support of partner also leads to feeling safe (oxytocin release).

Continue your mindfulness practice this week with a short activity (drinking your coffee, putting on makeup).

Create your own birth affirmations. Write them out and post them in places where you will see them 20 times a day. Start visualizing your perfect birth mind movie. You are the producer and director - this is your movie! Turn off the scary TV shows about birth.

▌HOW DO YOU KNOW LABOR HAS STARTED?

Just as with pregnancy, every woman experiences labor differently. In the weeks leading up to the birth, your baby may engage (move deeper into the pelvis) and you may have pre-labor warm-ups or surges that are helping your baby into the best position (these can sometimes be mistaken for the real thing). Even though it can be frustrating, your body is just preparing for the big day slowly and gently. Most GentleBirthing moms tend to start the birth process very gradually and easily not really sure if this is really it. Everything is happening for a reason.

Some women have loose bowel movements just prior to labor beginning or they feel as if they've eaten some questionable food. Sometimes moms have a burst of energy and feel the need to prepare their "nest," or a dull backache, often accompanied by a crampy premenstrual feeling. It can be tricky to pinpoint the actual start of labor because the buildup is often slow and gradual and sometimes takes place over a few days. Most women believe that labor starts with dilation but, in fact, there's a lot going on that moms aren't aware of before dilation can take place.

BIRTH STORY

"My baby arrived at 8pm exactly, 36 weeks, 4 lbs 2 oz. I went into spontaneous labor, I thought I had indigestion when I woke up that morning. I spent a few hours at home having breakfast and chatting with my parents, decided to go to hospital and check if all was ok about 1 pm. I had the trace and the heartbeat was fine. Then they performed an examination and I was fully effaced so they admitted me. My sister went and got us lunch and I asked for a ball as I didn't have anything like that with me. I sat on the ball and chatted with my sister and my husband came in around 3:30. I used the shower a few times, I had my birth preferences in a folder but had never discussed these with anyone. So talked them through with midwife. About 5:30, midwife asked if I would like to be examined again to consider moving to the delivery room. I said okay; after the examination we walked to the delivery room and on the way midwife asked was I doing GentleBirth. I used my breathing all the time and honestly felt relaxed and calm throughout. My waters went in the delivery room (naturally) and there was meconium so I had more monitoring. I delivered our little girl vaginally, tried gas and air in the delivery room but didn't like it. Labor couldn't have gone better! ....

Our baby girl was discharged last week so we are finally enjoying time at home and I'm delighted. Thank you, Bernie, for the class and for staying in touch. I found the last few weeks of pregnancy very stressful and the whole program really helped me to stay calm and focus on the positive. I'm so thrilled to have my gorgeous little girl here now."

HELPING YOUR BABY INTO THE BEST POSITION FOR BIRTH

Most babies settle into a particular position in the uterus during late pregnancy, called left occiput anterior or LOA. This position, in which the back of the baby's head points toward the mother's front and the baby's back is slightly to the left on the mother's side, is ideal, allowing for the easiest, safest, and quickest birth. Imagine this: Stand up and imagine your baby's head just above the pubic bone, your baby's back is along your left arm, and you'll feel kicks more toward the right. Check out spinningbabies.com for great tips and information on "bellymapping."

ENCOURAGING OPTIMAL POSITIONING

Imagine your belly button as a torch and we don't want the torch to shine on the ceiling for long periods in late pregnancy.

The baby's back is the heaviest side of its body. This means that the back will naturally gravitate toward the lowest side of the mother's abdomen. So if a mom's tummy is lower than her back, e.g. she is sitting on a chair leaning forward, then the baby's back will tend to swing toward her tummy. If the back is lower than her tummy, e.g. she is lying on her back or leaning back in an armchair, then the baby's back may swing toward the mother's back.

Avoid positions that encourage the baby to face your tummy. The main culprits are said to be lolling back in an armchair or a comfy couch, sitting in car seats where the mother is leaning back, or any position in which her knees are higher than her pelvis.

The best way to do this is to spend lots of time kneeling upright, sitting upright, or on hands and knees. When you sit on a chair, make sure your knees are lower than your pelvis, and the trunk should be tilted slightly forward.

Watch TV while kneeling on the floor, over a beanbag or cushions, or sit on a dining chair. Try sitting on a dining chair facing (leaning on) the back as well. Sit on a wedge cushion in the car.

Avoid sitting with your legs crossed. This reduces the space at the front of the pelvis and opens it up at the back. For good positioning, the baby needs to have lots of space at the front.

Avoid deep squatting, which opens up the pelvis and encourages the baby to move down, until it is known that the baby is the right way round.

Swimming with the belly downwards is great for positioning babies in utero. Moms who swim regularly report less back labor. Use lots of breaststroke and front crawl. Breaststroke, in particular, is thought to help with good positioning because all those leg movements help open the mom's pelvis and settle the baby downwards. A birth ball can encourage good positioning, both before and during labor.

Various exercises done on all fours can help, e.g., wiggling your hips from side to side, or arching your back like a cat, followed by dropping the spine down. Prenatal yoga can really help align your baby.

▌POSTERIOR LABOR

A small percentage of babies will remain in a posterior position during labor, which can make labor much more intense, especially in your back, and moms may also feel discomfort between surges. If you suspect your baby is in a posterior position, leaving your waters intact can help your baby rotate easier. Having a doula suggest position changes and comfort measures can make a big difference in how you experience your baby's birth especially with this kind of labor.

In labor, the all-fours position (backside in the air) may help your baby "back out" of the pelvis and come back down into a more favorable position. Firm pressure on the lower back by your partner or doula can be very helpful to deal with the discomfort of "back" labor.

On all fours, you can also lean over the birth ball. Put some pillows under your knees.

Straddle the toilet, facing backward (opening the pelvis).

Try abdominal lifting to change the 'drive angle': During a surge, place your hands beneath your abdomen and lift your abdomen gently while tilting your pelvis by bending your knees - this can help your baby get better aligned to enter the pelvis in a more favorable position.

A cold can from the fridge rolled on your lower back is a wonderful tool - even a rolling pin or tennis ball can be helpful to roll up and down the most uncomfortable area.

▌PROGRESS IS MORE THAN DILATION

Your cervix has kept your baby safe for 9 months so now lots of changes are happening to allow your baby a gentle exit. Your cervix moves from a posterior (pointing toward your back) to an anterior, more central position.

Your cervix ripens or softens; the consistency of an unripe cervix is like the feeling of the tip of your nose, hard, but when the cervix is ripe, it feels more like your lips, soft. Imagine the cervix melting like warm butter ... or soft chocolate.

- Your cervix effaces (shortens and thins).
- Your cervix begins to dilate and open.
- Your baby's head rotates, flexes (tucks his chin to chest), and compresses so the smallest diameter is coming first.
- Your baby descends, rotates more, and is born.

In most cases, the birth process won't start until both the baby and mom are ready for the birth. Electrical activity in the uterus causes the surges (triggered by oxytocin), so ideally both your brain and body are 'wired up' perfectly for a spontaneous start.

The usual ways to tell if labor has started are: there is a show; the waters release; and/or mom has surges that are regular and continue building in strength and become more frequent.

BIRTH

▌YOU HAVE A SHOW

Having a "show" refers to the release of bloodstained mucus as the cervix starts to thin and dilate. The show usually continues throughout labor and is a good sign of progress. The discharge is usually pink or red; if any amniotic fluid passes at the same time, it may also be a little blood-stained, but should then become clear. My general rule of thumb for first-time healthy moms considering when to go to the hospital or call your midwife is "no show - no go"!

However, if there is heavy bleeding or you're unsure about what's happening always contact your health care provider.

▌YOUR WATERS RELEASE

Sometimes labor can start with the release of your waters, that is, the amniotic fluid surrounding your baby releases, although sometimes the waters will not release until later in labor. The waters may also come out as a slow leak or trickle, where you may notice some dampness in your underwear, making it difficult to determine if it's amniotic fluid at all!

The waters are normally clear, but sometimes there is a little pink or red, which should become clear. If the waters are particularly red, there may be bleeding into the fluid; or, if they are brown or green, then the baby may have passed meconium. Contact your hospital or midwife immediately.

At this late stage of pregnancy, some mothers may leak a little urine. To determine if the leak is amniotic fluid or urine, the easiest way is to put on a pad – leave it for an hour and then do the sniff test - smell it; amniotic fluid is almost odorless and does not have a urine-like smell. However, if the smell is offensive, this might indicate an infection and your healthcare provider should be contacted immediately. Once your waters have released, the risk of infection increases. To minimize infection, you should avoid repeated vaginal exams. Bathing and showering in plain water do not increase the risk of infection.

It is useful to talk to your healthcare provider beforehand about their policy regarding what to do when the waters release and how long they are willing to wait for labor to start spontaneously. I was with a mom once who was told my the on call OB that once the waters release and labor hasn't started the uterus is like a 'burning building' and we need to 'get everyone out as quickly as possible'... hardly reassuring... Mom was well and declined kick starting her labor with Pitocin for 26 hours after her waters released and her surges began. Mom took her temperature every 4 hours and was happy to agree to medical intervention if she showed any signs of infection.

Some care providers may prefer you to go to the hospital immediately, while others are happy for the woman to stay at home for a while. The risk of infection is lower at home than at the hospital, so relax in the comfort of your own home while things get started.

If your baby is not yet at 37 weeks or is breech and the waters release, go to the hospital immediately.

THE SURGES ARE CONSISTENT AND SETTLE INTO A PATTERN

Moms often have Braxton-Hicks surges or tightenings for several days or weeks before the actual labor starts; they are irregular, they slow down or stop if you rest, and they have no proper pattern to them. Sometimes they will last for a few hours, surging every few minutes before stopping, which can be really frustrating. Think of these surges as warm-ups - just as you would warm up any other muscle before exercise. In this case, rest and conserve your energy, carry on with life as normal, or have a "labor project" to take your mind off the clock. While these practice, warm-up surges can be quite frustrating, they are in fact helping to soften and thin the cervix and just helping labor start gently. When the surges start to become longer, more intense, and closer together over time, showing a regular pattern, then this is a sign that true labor is underway.

Surges are usually felt as a wave, with a gentle start that increases to an intense peak before fading away gradually.

Initially, the surges may not feel particularly intense, more of a discomfort low down in the abdomen or back; they can be ignored or you can easily talk through them. They usually last for around 20-30 seconds at the start, increasing over time. They may occur at 20-30 minute intervals, increasing over time, or they can start straight away at 3-4 minute intervals. As labor progresses, you may need to focus more on each one, using slow rhythmic breathing to stay focused.

GOING TO THE HOSPITAL (STAY HOME UNTIL 4CM)

As the famous Clash song goes "should I stay or should I go now?" Timing the move to hospital is an important decision to make. Most moms labor better at home in the early stages because they feel more relaxed and comfortable in familiar surroundings, while others feel safer in the hospital right away; each mom and pregnancy is different. Partners will influence how comfortable you feel being at home longer. If your partner is wandering around the house jingling the car keys you won't feel very relaxed. For a low-intervention hospital birth, research recommends staying home longer to ensure that labor is well established before going into the hospital if you've had a healthy pregnancy. Moving to the hospital will sometimes slow down or stall things, which can then lead to interventions being needed to get things going again. Ask about your hospital guidelines. You'll know exactly when is the right time for you to go to the hospital or to call your midwife.

THE FLOW OF LABOR

Mainstream pregnancy guides tend to focus on labor being divided into distinct stages. However, there are no hard and fast segments of labor that become obvious as soon as you hit a certain number in dilation. Consider that labor is a continuum, a building of energy that is carrying you and your baby to your destination together.

EARLY SIGNS OF LABOR –
WHAT IS HAPPENING TO YOUR BODY?

The uterus will tighten and relax for "practice" or warm-up Braxton Hicks contractions, although some GentleBirth moms may not feel this. The cervix will change position (to an anterior position) and soften due to the release of hormones and may start to thin (efface), your waters may release. It's normal for the waters to release around 7-8cm. Your baby's head will engage and you may feel additional pressure in the pelvic region; this usually occurs earlier for first-time moms. In subsequent labors, your baby may not engage until well into labor.

WHAT ARE THE SIGNS?

You may feel backache or some Braxton Hicks surges or some tightenings.

Other early labor signs include a show, soft bowel movements, and nesting. Some women will experience pre-labor surges for a day or more: These are mild, frequent surges that may go on for a few hours before stopping. Most GentleBirth moms experience a gentle, gradual buildup and are usually already into a good rhythm of labor before they realize this is it and not just more warm-ups!

WHAT CAN YOU DO?

Relax, relax, and relax a bit more. Eat if you're hungry, particularly carbohydrates (rice, pasta, bread) for energy. Ditch the keto diet for labor. If you have a doula, update her on what is happening and how you are feeling. Try to go on doing normal things. This gentle, gradual buildup may last a day or more for a first-time mom, so try not to get too frustrated or excited. Keep a few movies handy that you've wanted to see. Resist the temptation to tell everyone you're in labor or you'll find yourself answering 50 text messages an hour from friends wondering if you've had your baby yet. Try not to update your Facebook page at this point but we'd love to support you in the private group!

WHAT IS HAPPENING TO YOUR BODY?

The cervix will efface (thin) and dilate (open) to 6cm (active labor); surges should be regular and start building up slowly in length and frequency.

WHAT ARE THE SIGNS?

Sometimes the waters release and the water comes out in a gush, you may have more show, or the surges may feel stronger and start to become more frequent. Labor surges should build up over the labor, generally lasting from 30 to 45 seconds at the start of labor to longer surges as your baby is being born. At this stage, the surges are usually between 3 minutes or as long as 20 minutes apart.

WHAT CAN YOU DO?

Rest, rest, rest. Have your birth partner keep a casual eye on the frequency of surges, Depending on the time of the day and how you feel, you may want to try to rest, eat (easily digested foods), or keep active between surges. Follow your body's lead. Make the environment as pleasant and relaxed as possible (think romance) allowing yourself to settle down emotionally and find your own rhythm, without any pressure to progress or perform.

ACTIVE LABOR - WHAT IS HAPPENING TO YOUR BODY?

Your cervix dilates from around 6cm to 10cm, your cervix opens more steadily and quickly than before, and surges become more powerful. Surges are regular and start building up slowly in length and frequency.

WHAT ARE THE SIGNS?

As surges get more intense, you will deepen your focus, taking long slow, deep rhythmic breaths.

WHAT CAN THE BIRTH PARTNERS DO?

Birth partners can time the surges, encourage mom to try different positions or movements such as walking, standing, rocking, swaying, slow dancing, squatting, kneeling, or side lying if tired. Mom - follow your body's lead, rest in between surges. Listen to the App. Get mom to focus on slow rhythmic breathing. Remind her to use the bathroom often to empty her bladder, and to try to snack, and stay relaxed. Focus on one surge at a time.

THE BIRTH OF YOUR BABY – WHAT IS HAPPENING TO YOUR BODY?

Depending on your body and baby, full dilation might be 9cm or 11cm. At this point, the nature of the surges changes. Sometimes the surges will disappear for a time, just to give your body a rest before the expulsive stage where your body nudges your baby down. With each surge, your baby moves downward slightly, then slips back up at the end of each surge.

The baby's head slowly stretches the vaginal tissue and the perineum, as you use focused breathing to breathe your baby down and go with your own urges so he emerges slowly. As the baby's head and then the body is born, it rotates.

WHAT ARE THE SIGNS?

When the baby has moved into the optimal position, most moms begin to feel a strong irresistible urge to breathe down or bear down, which becomes stronger and more frequent. The intensity feels "involuntary and uncontrollable." Your body is just doing it without you! The beginning of this phase can feel overwhelming as you get used to the power of nature moving through you. You have so much happening in your pelvis, so many intense sensations... ligaments are stretching, your pelvis is shifting and your baby is moving through you.

WHAT CAN YOUR BIRTH PARTNER DO?

Keep mom relaxed and remind her to focus on her breathing. Apply a warm compress to the perineal area to soften and relax the area for mom and to reduce the risk of perineal injury.

Encourage mom to use a position comfortable to her (upright, on hands and knees, supported squat, kneeling, standing, or, if the mom is tired side lying), and take it nice and slowly as the head emerges.

THIRD STAGE—BIRTH OF THE PLACENTA

After your baby is born, he will continue to receive oxygenated and nutrient-rich blood from the placenta for several minutes. Up to 30% of your baby's blood gets trapped in the placenta if the cord is clamped prematurely and the placenta amputated. Allowing the cord to finish pulsating for even five minutes has significant benefits for your baby. Leaving the cord alone gives your baby time to adapt to using his lungs for the first time and receives iron that reduces his risk of anemia.

You may feel uterine cramps as opposed to strong surges, although the after-birth sensations with subsequent children are often stronger.

THE FOURTH STAGE—THE GOLDEN HOUR

Enjoy these first few magical moments. Your baby may or may not be interested in feeding right away; your baby knows what to do. Keep your baby warm with as much skin-to-skin contact (naked on your chest) as possible and uninterrupted time together. Your baby has just moved house very suddenly. Skin-to-skin contact calms your baby's stress response, keeps him at the perfect temperature and regulates his breathing and blood sugars. This is a massive time of brain changes for both you and your baby as your brain floods with oxytocin, which is "switching on" your maternal brain. Just like your new baby, there is also an "unfolding" of your new maternal brain. There's no need for your baby to wear a hat during your skin-to-skin time. As your brain switches gears, it needs to "breathe in your baby" to help turn on the mothering center of the brain. Moms and babies can recognize each other through smell alone. All mammals lick their babies after birth; this instinctive action has an important function. We don't lick our babies but kiss them quite compulsively. As you kiss your baby your brain is being given instructions on the perfect composition of the milk for your baby. Skin to skin with your baby flat on your body triggers your baby's feeding behaviors so lie back and enjoy your new baby while he settles in.

THE LABOR RECIPE

Your bags are packed and sitting in the hall....the floors are gleaming and everything is ready. The stack of well-read pregnancy books sits on the kitchen table with highlighted sections for your partner. After lots of research and stories from friends, you're determined not to be one of those women who panic at the first strange tightening sensation of labor and race off to the hospital, only to find out to their mortification that it was just trapped wind.

First labors are such a unique experience and, even after reading every pregnancy book on the planet, you're still not quite sure what to expect.

Thankfully, there is quite a lot you and your partner can do together at home to make this time at home before you go into the hospital memorable and comfortable. Dr. Michel Odent, the French obstetrician who pioneered the birth pool, has some suggestions for creating the conditions for a shorter, easier labor and what he refers to as an "undisturbed birth." Dr. Sarah Buckley has also written extensively on the topic of ecstatic birth and the perfect blend of birth hormones in her book *Gentle Birth, Gentle Mothering*.

There are two ways to "blend" this cocktail of hormones in labor:

- By medically managing them (giving mom artificial hormones to chemically drive her surges, such as Pitocin).
- By "hacking" your natural hormones by using the techniques in this program.

Which do you think will be easiest on your body and on your baby?

Here are some suggestions to encourage a natural release of birth hormones designed perfectly for your body and your baby that come only with positive side effects.

- You need to feel safe and uninhibited. If you feel stressed and anxious, your body releases adrenaline, which is the brake of labor. When you feel safe and not afraid, your body produces oxytocin and endorphins, which are labor helpers. When you feel uninhibited, you can easily slip into the primal part of your mind that regulates that perfect hormonal blend.
- You need to feel unobserved, so don't text or call everyone that your labor has started. You'll be plagued by well-meaning friends and family and you'll start to suffer from a kind of labor performance anxiety; you'll begin to think that you're taking too long (your mental meerkat will be activated).
- Dim lighting. Get your candles out and hit the dimmer switch. Bright fluorescent lighting inhibits the hormonal release by interrupting the production of melatonin, which is a helper hormone for oxytocin. Bono rockstar sunglasses aren't uncommon for GentleBirth moms.
- Excessive conversation also keeps you in your reasoning and analytical part of your mind, so rest and use your brain training. Activating the language center of the brain means valuable resources are being used up unnecessarily.

Keep activity low, both mentally and physically. Despite what you might have read, Olympic speed walking in early labor is unhelpful UNLESS it feels good to do so. Don't walk for miles because someone told you to or because you read it online. High activity inhibits your helper hormones and increases adrenaline, plus you want to conserve as much energy as you can. Rest, rest, rest.

OXYTOCIN BOOST TECHNIQUE

Close your eyes and think of someone who really, really loves and cares about you - it could be a parent your partner maybe even a family pet? Let all of those wonderful memories come up for a few moments. By remembering a time of feeling loved and cared about, the brain releases oxytocin, which, as you know by now, is the antidote to adrenaline.

I know it's a bit of a stretch for first-time moms and dads to associate labor with romance, so bear with me. I can already hear the ewwwwwws as you read this. But if you look at it scientifically, it's the same perfect cocktail of hormones that resulted in most moms becoming pregnant that helps your baby to be born.

Just look back at the points above - feeling safe, uninhibited, unobserved, with dim lighting and not much conversation might remind you of when you were dating your partner and the things you did to create a romantic atmosphere and get in the mood. You see where I'm going? The more intimate and, yes, romantic the environment you can create at home, the more likely your labor is to progress quicker and easier.

Even your partner's sexy hypnotic voice has a role to play in getting your baby out (after all, for most moms, it was your partner's sexy hypnotic voice that helped get the baby there in the first place).

Have a labor project that requires low mental and physical activity. Put on the App and sleep if you can.

Watch a funny movie. Laughter releases endorphins, your labor helpers. Endorphins give you a sense of wellbeing (like the high you get from chocolate).

Bake a birthday cake for your baby.

Your partner can run you a warm bath and light the candles add some lavender essential oil, which also has a pain-relieving effect on the body. Labor in warm water as much as possible to promote oxytocin release.

Water immersion during the birth process is a must. If you don't have a deep bath, you can purchase a birth pool online and labor in it before going to the hospital. Moms who labor in water tend to have quite short birth experiences (five hours for a first-time mom).

Your partner can cook you some nice food and encourage you to stay hydrated with water, soup, or isotonic drinks (coconut water is great).

Have a relaxing massage or foot rub (with clary sage, lavender, or rose essential oils).

Your partner can put on some nice music, any easy listening music that has positive memories for you.

He/she can make sure there is gas in the car and not panic when it's time to go.

Ask your partner to read this or play it for them if you're listening to the book.

Unless he's been to a GentleBirth Class he probably hasn't read all those highlighted pages you've prepared for him just yet and probably won't. His eyes may move across the pages but his mind is most likely on the football results.

"The parallels between making love and giving birth are clear, not only in terms of passion and love, but also because we need essentially the same conditions for both experiences: privacy and safety."
–Sarah Buckley–

▌EMERGENCY CHILDBIRTH

Over the years there have been a few GentleBirth babies born unexpectedly on the way to the hospital or at home. All of the babies were born quickly and without any complications and the moms were ecstatic (not exactly what people generally expect as a 'positive' birth experience').

So you think baby is coming NOW and you've made the decision not to get in the car and fight the Friday evening traffic ... (or there's been a zombie apocalypse and there are no hospitals!).

First off - healthy babies pretty much deliver themselves - your partner's job is to remain calm and gently catch.

Don't freak out; call the paramedics and/or your midwife.

Unlatch the front door so the paramedics can let themselves in.

In winter, boost up the heating and grab some blankets.

Stay with your partner and reassure her (trust me on this one - we can smell fear).

As your baby's head emerges, hold your hands just under baby's head. You do not have to pull on your baby's head.

Encourage your partner to breathe slowly and deeply and resist the urge to push. Mom's body will push baby out.

As the rest of your baby's body emerges, simply support him with your hands as you reassure your partner.

Gently lift your baby to mom's chest for immediate skin-to-skin and cover mom and baby with blankets. Skin-to-skin regulates baby's temperature and breathing.

No need to touch the cord no shoelaces no zip ties...or twist ties. The cord will continue to give your baby oxygen as it pulsates for the next several minutes.

Remove any wet towels/blankets from baby and replace with dry ones.

If the placenta comes out just leave it next to mom.

Breathe - help is on the way.

ROADSIDE BIRTH

If you're in the car, calmly pull over with your hazard lights on and call an ambulance.

Turn up the heat in the car.

Help your partner remove her underwear/trousers.

Reassure your partner by staying calm (even if you're screaming on the inside).

Gently receive baby into your hands - no pulling on baby's head.

Place baby skin-to-skin with mom and cover with any blankets/clothes you have available.

Leave the cord alone as above and await help (it's normal for baby to be a bit blue initially; healthy babies pink up very quickly).

If baby arrives quickly, he/she may be a little shocked at the speed with which he just 'moved house'. If baby seems to be a bit stunned, simply rub baby's back and/or tap the soles of baby's feet.

BIRTH STORY

I woke up on the morning of my due date to mild period-like pain, I felt excited but also very aware that this could be something or nothing. I had a lie-in and tried to forget about the surge that I had felt and decided to just enjoy my day and see what it brought. As the day progressed I continued to have irregular mild surges. We had a lovely time, taking Orla to feed the ducks, eating lunch together and relaxing. As the day went on the surges became a little bit more frequent - roughly every 30 mins but I could still hold a conversation throughout them. I was really happy to be able to rest between surges as when I had Orla I had little or no break in between so this was proving to be a very different labor with a completely different pattern. Throughout the evening I chatted to my mom about looking after Orla should I need to go to hospital. I laid out her clothes for the next day, I changed her bedsheets, organised her dinner and breakfast for the following morning and gave her lottos kisses and cuddles, all this helped me feel organized and in control of the situation - it was lovely knowing that I didn't have to worry about Orla and that she would be very well cared for when I needed to make the move.

My mom decided she would like my niece to come over and help with Orla, so my sister-in-law dropped my niece over, it was really surreal chatting calmly though surges, joking about what lay ahead and I remember telling my sister-in-law that this time around I would really love to avoid an epidural if at all possible but that I was open to what ever came our way.

At around 6pm I noticed that I needed to concentrate a little harder during the surges but they were very manageable and simply closing my eyes and breathing through them was enough. We had our usual nighttime routine, Paul gave Olivia a bath and we said good night to her and put her to bed. I remember feeling a little bit melancholy as I walked out of her room, knowing that it was likely that the next day she would no longer be my baby. After Olivia was put to bed I had a shower and settled down to have an oxytocin filled night, I watched Downton Abbey while Paul went to get me my favorite takeout. By the time he came home the surges were more regular about 8-10 minutes apart, but still very manageable. I remember feeling really calm and happy to be able to rest between surges, it was really lovely to quietly anticipate the arrival of our baby in such a fear free way. We watched some feel good TV. At around 9.30pm Paul rang the hospital to let them know that labor had begun and that if possible we would like to use the pool if it was free. The midwife informed us that it would probably be a while before we would need to come in, and that they had someone in the birthing suite at that point. We decided at around 10.30pm to go to bed and try and get some rest. Paul made sure that everything we needed was in the car and I laid out everything that I would need for making the transition into the hospital.

We went to bed and fell asleep (I was really surprised that I could sleep but also very relieved) every time I had a surge we would time the contraction. I was mainly lying on my side and I found that breathing deeply and slowly and rocking from side to side helped me to stay focused during the surges. Paul repeated my affirmations to me and reassured me with every surge. It was lovely being in our own environment with nobody else there and feeling able to ask Paul to speak to me more slowly and to speak up when I couldn't hear him through a surge - we had put so much effort and planning into working as a team for this birth, it felt like everything was falling into place and that we were working together as our baby was getting ready to be born.

I remember going to the toilet a few times and expecting to see a show but there was no sign of anything, I remember looking at the clock and thinking by 3am I think I will be in active labor.

When I stood up to go to the bathroom I felt the pressure and surges were much more intense, so I was more comfortable lying on my side in the comfort of the bed, I still can't believe that I was able to sleep in-between surges, I had heard about people doing this before but I didn't think it was true. I remember saying to myself that my body wouldn't make a surge that I couldn't handle and that I could handle anything for a minute. Paul was repeating these affirmations to me throughout the surges also, so I had nothing but positive thoughts coming my way. At 2am I vomited, and thought that maybe things were beginning to happen, but I honestly felt that if I had gone to the hospital at that stage they would have told me I was only a few centimeters dilated. At around 3am I had a couple of very intense surges, it was the first time that I felt that I needed to reach out and hold Paul's hand, I really felt that I needed him beside me at that point, and during those few surges I experienced a little bit of self doubt and fear and I remember telling Paul that I really needed him and that I couldn't do it. Paul reassured me, repeating my affirmations to me, and it was like a switch flicking in my head and I remember feeling filled with determination and positivity and smiling and saying 'I can do this, I am doing this, I can do this...' it was at that moment that I knew that I would be able to deliver my baby naturally, I was filled with calmness and I just knew that I would do it.

Paul suggested that we make a move to the hospital but at that point the surges were coming very regularly and I had to wait for a few to pass before I felt able to stand up. Paul ran downstairs to give my mom the baby monitor. When he came back, I got up and started to get ready. At this point the surges were coming so fast that Paul could hardly get my shoe on before I had to jump back onto the bed on all fours and breathe through the surge. We made our way downstairs and my mom was there to give me a hug and tell me that she loved me before we left, when we got to the front door I remember saying to myself "this baby is coming" as I breathed through another surge.

We walked to the car and when I got to the car door I felt an extremely intense urge to push, all the while I was feeling very calm and in control, I remember telling Paul to go ahead and get into the car and that I would get in once the surge passed. I remember saying to Paul as I felt the urge to push "this is bigger than me" - I had heard about the intensity of the urge to push before, but it was only at that point that I realized just how powerful and beyond my control it was. Paul reassured me that I was probably feeling the pressure of my waters about to go, but that we should start moving. Paul rang the hospital to let them know that we were on our way, while he was talking to the midwife my waters released and the urge to push intensified. The midwife advised Paul that the baby was coming in a hurry and not to delay. Paul asked me did I want to go to another hospital because it was closer and I remember saying no because a part of me didn't want to admit that the baby was going to be born so soon. Up until the point where my waters released I had hoped the urge to push might ease off and we would have time to reach the hospital but the surges intensified along with the urge to push and as we joined the M50 I told Paul pull in "this is happening now, call an ambulance." Paul pulled in on the hard shoulder and rang 999. I remember hearing the emergency responder talk to him, and being able to answer a few of the questions myself, I thought "I cant believe this is happening here" but I knew that I was powerless to stop the baby from coming as the urge to push intensified and overtook my body.

Paul took off my shoes and pyjama bottoms and put down the passenger seat as far as it could go, as I felt the need to turn over onto all fours. I remember the emergency responder reminding me to breathe, and seeing the flashing lights as the fire brigade pulled up beside the car. The next thing that I remember is the burning sensation of the baby's head crowning and feeling somebody putting their hand on the area, I thought it was Paul and I remember shouting for him to take his hands off me as I felt it was preventing the baby from being born, it was actually a paramedic and he reassured me that he was trying to help me as the baby was being born so fast. I remember feeling reassured by this and remembering that he was protecting my perineum as the baby's head emerged.

I remember calling out to Paul saying that I needed him, and he reassured me that he was right beside me at the car door. As the baby's head was born I felt a massive relief, I remember being able to rest my chest and stomach on the back of the seat and breathing as I waited for the baby's body to be born, already I was feeling elated. Our baby shot into the world, summersaulting on her way out into the hands of the paramedic at 3.45am, a mere 15 minutes after we had left the house.

I asked Paul what the baby was and he said I think it's a girl, and the paramedics confirmed that we had a daughter. I asked for delayed cord clamping, but as the paramedics thought that I was hemorrhaging they told me that they couldn't delay clamping the cord but they let Paul do the honors. The paramedics seemed concerned about the amount of blood I was loosing and this was the first time that I felt fear, I remember thinking "I can't die after doing that!" They reassured me and helped me to step out of the car and onto a stretcher as they transferred me into the ambulance, everything at this point is a bit hazy but I remember getting to hold our baby girl, seeing her little purple feet and her dark hair and feeling totally elated, shocked and in love.

The paramedics gave the baby to Paul to hold while they did what they had to with me, as we were transferred to the hospital I was desperate to hold the baby but the paramedic explained to me that he had to hold her for her safety but ensured that I could see her for the whole journey. It was a really surreal journey, I remember almost not being able to look at the baby as I couldn't quite believe what had just happened. When we got to the hospital the baby was taken to the delivery suite ahead of me to be warmed up. I was brought into the same room and welcomed by lovely midwives. Paul arrived and stayed with the baby while the midwives looked after me. The paramedics expressed concern that I had lost a lot of blood after the baby was born but the midwives didn't at all seem concerned and reassured me that everything seemed fine. Before the paramedics left we made sure that the baby had her photo taken with them and I remember as they left feeling the urge to tell them that I loved them as they had done such an amazing job and witnessed such a momentous occasion in our lives. We assured them that we would call into them at their station for them to see the baby again.

After the paramedics had left, the midwife helped me to deliver the placenta, I was so happy to be able to do this naturally as this was part of my birth preferences. After the placenta had been delivered I was given Syntocinon as there had been a concern about a postpartum hemorrhage. The midwife examined me and seemed confident that I hadn't been damaged too much, then a doctor arrived to examine me, she was concerned that I may have had a 3rd degree tear but as I was so tender we agreed that she could take a closer look and do whatever repair was necessary with a spinal anaesthetic. At this point I was very happy to agree to that as the baby had been safely delivered and I was tired and sore and didn't want to feel any further discomfort. I got to hold and feed the baby for a good half hour and we decided to name her Alanna. After giving her a feed and having skin to skin, I handed her over to her daddy for a snooze and more skin to skin cuddles while I went down to theatre to get stitched up. Luckily I managed to avoid a third degree tear and I was back holding little Alanna within 45 minutes. After that, our baby-moon began, we had tea and toast and marvelled at our gorgeous daughter and all that had happened.

I can honestly say that the prospect of having our baby at the side of the road would have terrified me but it was honestly the most wonderful, positive, fear free experience of my life. Apart from a couple of shaky moments as I transitioned, I honestly felt no fear throughout the whole labor and birth. Affirmations, surrounding myself with positive stories, listening to GentleBirth tracks, and doing everything possible to boost my oxytocin levels all helped me to achieve the birth that I wanted. Having my amazing husband support me in preparing Alanna's birth was wonderful and I couldn't have done it without his support throughout the whole journey; I felt unconditionally supported and I could not imagine a more wonderful birth partner or father to our girls.

Our little baby is now three weeks old, feeding beautifully, sleeping soundly and filling our lives with love and joy. Despite her somewhat speedy arrival, she has been calm and content from the beginning, we have no doubt that her birth story will be told every year on her birthday with joy and pride and love.

BIRTH BLESSING

by Natalie Evans

Close your eyes and breathe deep
Breathe in peace, breathe out pain
Imagine your feet
Toes curling into dirt
Think of yourself as rooted
Think of your place in the earth
How did you come to be here?
Through generations of women named
A maternal lineage
That brought you to this place
Think of their birth stories
What you know, what you believe to be true Realize that their births carry deep wisdom
Some may carry the memory of joy and transcendence
Each birth is a powerful experience
Each birth traces down to you.
Just as you pass this knowledge on to your baby
Understand that your birth is your own
It will be different from all others
Like the swirls in your thumb
Your birth will have a unique pattern
Unfolding with each surge
Rising and falling like a newborn's chest
This birth belongs to you
This birth is an opening
This birth is the end and a beginning
May this blessing of birth come to you without fear
May this blessing of birth come to you with great understanding May this blessing of birth make your heart soar
May this blessing of birth bring shouts of delight to your lips
Blessings to you and your birth.

BIRTH PLANS, PREFERENCES AND PRIORITIES

> "Prepare for a no fault birth....If you confidently participate in all the decisions made during your labor and delivery - even those that were not in your birth plan - you are likely to look upon your birth with no blame and no regrets."
>
> William and Martha Sears - The Birth Book

One of the most important skills needed by a new parent is the ability to make decisions. Every pregnant mom is faced with a million choices and often conflicting information. Every couple with a newborn finds that they are essentially "on their own" after the new baby arrives. That's why learning the skill of sound decision making now is key.

BIRTH PRIORITIES

Birth plans/preferences are essential if you want to avoid routine procedures. Some women advise not to do them based on their own experiences of having a birth plan. You may hear, "Don't make a birth plan because then you have high expectations and you can't control everything and you'll be disappointed, etc., etc." Maybe we should have high expectations for the biggest day of our lives? Your hospital has a birth plan for you so shouldn't you explore what that plan is and if it aligns with your vision of a positive birth?

Writing a birth plan is in some ways like preparing for a vacation or any other big event: It's all about planning and knowing what to expect and being prepared for all eventualities. You first need to know where it is that you want to go, followed by how you are going to get there and the things that you will need while you are there and what you plan to do while on holiday.

If your best friend told you not to make a wedding plan and told you to just go with the flow and let the wedding planner (or your mother-in-law) take care of everything, how would you respond?

You wouldn't just NOT make solid wedding plans just because you can't control the weather... you would have a contingency plan... a plan B......

you're getting married in July... and you want an outside champagne reception when the guests arrive from the church. Well, you'd find a hotel that offered that service and you'd discuss a backup plan with them just in case it rains. You can't control the weather but, if you'd chosen a hotel without the option of moving the reception inside, then you'd have a very different experience and most likely a very disappointing one.

We can't control everything in birth but you can explore all your options so you're the one in the driver's seat. There is lots you can control and you can always control your reaction to what's going on around you.

You're asking questions and hopefully getting the answers you want that are in line with your dream wedding. In some circumstances, planning a GentleBirth requires the same commitment and attention.

▌DO I NEED BIRTH PREFERENCES?

I definitely recommend considering writing a couple of points but it depends on you and your partner. How involved do you want to be regarding decisions being made about your care in the hospital?

Some women prefer to completely go with the flow and hope that everything will turn out fine and others want to be involved and included in any decisions that may affect them or their baby. Of course, there are rare circumstances when deferring to the medical expert opinion is necessary but, considering that almost 80 - 90% of women have straightforward pregnancy and births, it's unlikely that this will be the case for you. The key word here is "involved" and, in the context of labor, you could define that as having a curious attitude about routine offerings at your hospital.

For some hospitals, it means policies have been implemented involving routine procedures to help speed things up without it being clinically necessary.

Think of your birth plan as your birth preferences, birth priorities, or an expression of your expectations. Even if you never write them down, it's a good discussion starter with your midwife/obstetrician on how you'd like to be supported during your baby's birth. Chances are you'll have never met your midwife before, so it helps her understand what's important to you. Keep your preferences flexible, depending on what's going on during your baby's birth.

Sometimes it can just help you get your thoughts organized about what you'd like or not like ahead of time, along with understanding what you're likely to be offered at your hospital. You also have a chance ahead of time to consider what your options are if things don't go as planned. This often gives couples a sense of relief that they know they can handle whatever comes their way during the birth of their baby.

Some moms shy away from writing down their birth preferences, especially if they have the mistaken belief that it's going to guarantee that specific things will or won't happen during labor; we know that babies don't read birth plans.

There aren't any guarantees in labor so, if you are expecting that a birth plan is going to guarantee that something will or won't happen, then you could really be setting yourself up for disappointment. It's not the birth plan itself that can cause disappointment in labor but your expectations and motivation for creating it.

Sometimes I will hear moms who say, "As soon as I got to the hospital the birth plan went out the window." If you've done your homework, have prepared well, and you understand the offerings at your hospital in managing your labor, then this is highly unlikely to happen as you and your partner are making all of the decisions with input from your midwife/obstetrician - and not the other way around.

WHAT DOES THE RESEARCH SAY?

I was really excited to read a recent study that suggests birth preferences and attending birth preparation classes significantly reduce cesarean births in first-time mothers.

The study included over 20,000 births in the Los Angeles area and suggests that first time mothers who attended childbirth education and had written birth preferences were significantly more likely to have a vaginal birth (72.6% vs. 64.1%).

Even more encouraging is Amy DeBaets 2017 AJOG (Call to Action) for care providers to move away from hospital 'checklist' style birth plans to 'birth partnership' discussions throughout pregnancy so there is open communication between mother and care provider and if there are significant differences in ethos there is plenty of time for discussion and informed decision making.

Consider taking a GentleBirth workshop so you'll learn what's available in your place of birth and understand more about how to effectively write and communicate your preferences. Whenever possible talk through your wishes with your care provider (bring your partner along too) long before your EDD.

AVOIDING WOBBLES AT BIRTH PREFERENCE DISCUSSIONS

When speaking to your care provider about your birth preferences in pregnancy, remember to use the two questions if you find the discussion stressful. This will help keep the fear response on a tight leash so you can gather more information to help you make an informed decision.

Question 1 - What is my brain telling me right now?

Question 2 - Is it useful?

New research recommends a few moments of meditation before any medical appointment. Just a few minutes listening to the App before your appointment will help you retain more information and feel calmer to ask questions.

SAMPLE SCENARIO

You're 39 weeks after a near-perfect pregnancy. However your baby is not engaged and is predicted to be a 'big' baby. Your care provider has just suggested that you induce an induction or planned cesarean. If you've been attending your appointments with the expectation of a spontaneous labor supported by your care provider this out of the blue recommendation can throw up a huge wobble.

Right now, your brain is probably throwing up all kinds of worst-case scenarios of what this unengaged baby means for the length of your labor, your perineum, and your pain tolerance.

Are those thoughts useful? Nope! Not even a bit – especially as we don't make good decisions when the 'college' students are in charge. We need to create that bit of distance between the brain and you so you don't jump on an unfortunate train of thought to terror town.

Now you can calmly and rationally respond to your care provider "Thank you, Dr. Graham, we will consider this carefully and let you know our decision".

GentleBirth Mom

"GentleBirth gave me autonomy. It was a wonderful experience. I have children and only learned about it for my last labor. I would highly recommend it. I labored alone with my player and my TENS machine. I felt very much in control. I recommend to anyone who will listen to me."

HOSPITAL PROCEDURES - ROUTINE OR RARE?

Time Limits on Labor

At the time of publishing the WHO published new research that recommends re-evaluating the time limits on labor. You might be surprised to learn that in some hospitals you are on the clock. There is an outdated expectation that your cervix will dilate at 1cm per hour and if it doesn't then your uterus must be dysfunctional (instead of considering the guideline could be dysfunctional). Thankfully the start of active labor is now considered 6cm which means there's no need to accelerate your labor before then – but it's still very common. Talk to your careprovider about the average length of labor for a healthy first time mom – 24 hours wouldn't be unusual.

EATING IN LABOR - WHY IT'S GOOD FOR YOU AND YOUR BABY

As a mom-to-be, you've probably never been more focused on food than any other time in your life. Even analogies about baby's size and our body parts are associated with food, as if we weren't obsessed enough! Your baby is the size of a bean... your uterus is now the size of a grapefruit your boobs are like well, you get the picture! You've probably spent endless hours online researching what you can and can't eat during pregnancy.

Some moms have cravings and can't get enough of a particular food, while others struggle with all-day morning sickness and it takes a huge amount of willpower and determination to even get a few dry crackers past your lips.

There's also pica, which is the term for unusual cravings. The reason that some women develop pica cravings during pregnancy is not known for certain. There is currently no identified cause; but, according to the Journal of American Dietetic Association, there may be a connection to an iron deficiency.

Some speculate that pica cravings are the body's attempt to obtain vitamins or minerals that are missing from a mom's diet.

The most common substances craved during pregnancy are dirt/clay. Other pica cravings include burnt matches, stones, charcoal, mothballs, ice, cornstarch, toothpaste, soap, sand, plaster, coffee grounds, baking soda, and cigarette ashes...... ewwwwww!

A balanced diet in pregnancy is essential for both mom and baby. Expectant moms often spend a significant amount of time "grazing" or snacking regularly to keep their blood sugar normal.

If you've missed a meal lately, you've probably experienced some of the following side effects:

Increased crankiness

Exhaustion due to low blood sugar. You may even have passed out.

Skipping meals during pregnancy isn't recommended and you'd never willingly starve yourself during your pregnancy, so why would you do it in labor?

Let's look at the history of where this began and what can happen when a mom is refused nourishment during labor (assuming she's hungry).

Mendelson's Syndrome: This refers to the inhalation of gastric contents of the stomach and is a risk during intubation for a general anesthetic (you've probably seen intubation on "Grey's Anatomy").

Today most cesareans are performed with a spinal or epidural. It is rare to have a general anesthetic for a cesarean birth. The original article by Mendelson dates back to 1946, so it's a little bit outdated. The great news is that in 1961 a technique called Sellick's maneuver was developed, which minimized the risk of gastric contents entering the lungs during a general anesthetic.

What a breakthrough for laboring moms. It meant that all normal low-risk women (80 - 90% of moms reading this) could go back to eating in labor again!! Yay!!! But wait a minute that was over 47 years ago obviously some hospitals missed that memo.

Without food for a long period of time, a laboring mom's body enters into ketosis. When you first deprive your body of food, your metabolism begins to shift to accommodate this. The first stage is known as lipolysis, which means your body is burning fat to provide you with energy (sounds like a great way of burning off those extra pregnancy pounds...... AFTER you've had your baby!!)

Ketosis is the second part of the process that takes place when your body has no carbs to provide it with energy so it needs to use the energy from the fat being burned; in a nutshell (see, can't stay away from those food analogies). The unused portions of the fat cells are called ketones and are removed from the body in the urine. Ketosis is a signal that you are breaking down your fat reserves...... your body is effectively eating itself to give you energy during labor.

So you're at the hospital ... starving ... snappy ... exhausted and that's just your partner! Plus you feel pain much more intensely. That doesn't sound like a recipe for a positive birth.

Of course, some moms have no interest in eating in labor, if they're very anxious and afraid during labor, adrenaline slows the digestive process.

If you're giving birth in a hospital that is stuck back in the 1940s, bring along some snacks for yourself and your partner - just in case you do get hungry. Chances are you won't be in the mood for a Big Mac.

Thankfully there are some fantastic midwives around that are happy for you to snack to keep your energy levels up if you're hungry, so all is not lost.

Bon appétit!!

BIRTH PLANS AND FINE DINING

If you've attended some hospital prenatal classes, you will have had the set menu or what I call the drive-thru menu explained to you. What you probably don't know is that your hospital has a wonderful a la carte menu available too. You'd probably stop going to your favorite restaurant if they suddenly changed the menu and took all of your favorites off because the drive-thru menu was quicker and more cost-effective for the restaurant.

WHAT'S ON THE DRIVE-THRU MENU?

- Frequent vaginal exams to make sure you haven't deviated from the set timetable.
- Your waters are artificially released to speed up the process.
- IV Pitocin to speed up your labor if you don't keep up with the hospital timetable.
- Continuous monitoring (making it much harder to move about) and a very high false positive rate of detecting distress babies.

- Epidural needed due to the IV Pitocin which has made the surges more intense for you and your baby.
- Cesarean or forceps/vacuum to pull your baby out when the epidural affects pushing and your time is up.
- Episiotomy from the assisted delivery.

(Note: If you choose the set menu above you may only have 12 hours or less to give birth.)

GIVING BIRTH A LA CARTE

As with any dining experience, you decide what appeals to you and, if you're not sure, then having a helpful midwife recommend an option to you can be priceless. She may suggest options to you that you might never have considered before to make your experience a good one.

Assuming that all things are normal, there's no hurry, no time limits. You can choose not to have the drip and labor in your own time and on your terms. You may decide that releasing the waters so early isn't for you. Midwives are experts in a la carte birth and are great resources in helping you choose what's right for you and your baby, rather than the drive-thru menu that everyone else gets.

That's why putting some thought into what you want in labor is so important. Having the drive-thru menu just because it's all you've been offered often results in more intervention than is necessary and not as positive an experience. Yes, you'll probably have your baby quicker (drive-thru is all about speed and convenience), but your experience may not be as positive as it would have been had you known the wonderful a la carte options that were available. A la carte births are usually easier to achieve at home (after all, you own the restauran.) or at a birth center.

You can, of course, choose to have the drive-thru menu. If speed is your main priority and you'd rather have someone choose the menu for you, then drive-thru can be very appealing. Having no idea of what you want and choosing to just go with the flow means you let the staff choose the menu for you; that's exactly what you want if there is an emergency ... they are the experts ... but as most women have normal labors, a la carte is generally the safest way to go for you and your baby. International studies have also shown that the drive-thru menu is not the healthiest option for moms and babies.

Get thinking about your choices and how you can make this experience as positive as possible. Once you're in the line for drive-thru, it's tricky to get out of it. You just follow the car ahead of you and hope for the best. Comparing birth to a fine dining experience may be a stretch, but ask yourself: Do you want a drive-thru delivery, where you get what you're given (physically healthy baby and hopefully a physically healthy mom) or the a la carte birth, where it's about safety and quality (yes, you can have both ...... mom and

baby are both physically and emotionally healthy... I know what Gordon Ramsay would say...)

SAMPLE BIRTH PRIORITIES

My partner and I are looking forward to having a positive birth experience at _____ with your support.

We understand that birth can be unpredictable but if my baby and I are well we would appreciate your support in the following areas.

During Labor

- I would like to keep vaginal exams to a minimum (i.e., on admission) and only at my request after that (unless there is a concern for my baby).
- I prefer not to have an IV or hep-lock on admission.
- I prefer to labor and birth in any position that I find comfortable.
- I prefer to have intermittent monitoring unless there is a concern for my baby.
- As long as labor progresses normally and my baby and I are well, I prefer not to have my waters released or have my labor speeded up with Pitocin.
- When I am fully dilated, and assuming our baby is doing well, I would like to wait until I feel the urge to push before beginning the second stage.
- If I have an epidural I prefer to have at least 1-2 hours of passive descent before beginning active pushing.
- I prefer not to have an episiotomy.
- I prefer that my baby does not have routine suctioning if all is well.
- If all is well I prefer to have a physiological 3rd stage.

After the Birth

- If my labor has minimal intervention I prefer a physiological third stage.
- Please allow the cord to finish pulsating and wait until it is white.

- I would prefer to have immediate uninterrupted skin-to-skin with my baby.
- I prefer for my baby not to have antibiotic eye ointment as I have been tested in pregnancy for STDs.
- Please delay all non-urgent routine procedures such as weighing, Vitamin K, and baby checks.
- I plan to breastfeed.

SPECIAL CIRCUMSTANCES

Should intervention become necessary, we would appreciate being fully informed of all risks, benefits, and alternatives.

If a cesarean becomes necessary, my partner will remain with me at all times. Time permitting, I prefer not to have general anesthesia and would like to have the drape lowered to see my baby being born and have immediate skin-to-skin.

BIRTH STORY

First-Time Mom's Experience

On Sunday, I was convinced that I would have my baby the following day (my EDD was the Saturday). I went for a lovely walk in the park and felt the pressure of my baby in my pelvis but no surges or any pain, just an overall 'sense' (possibly wishful thinking!). The head had been engaged since week 38 so I had thought I would not go too far over the EDD. I had a disturbed night's sleep on Sunday night but I am a heavy sleeper so it could have been surges, I don't know! Monday morning 8am I had a show and started to feel surges irregularly. I told my husband it would probably be a good idea for him to stay off work and come with me to my consultant's appointment I had that morning at 11. The consultant listened to what I was feeling and told me I could be a few days away or imminent and offered to check if I wished. I accepted and she was quite surprised to inform me that I was fully effaced and 3-4cm dilated. Since I am quite near to the Coombe, she suggested I head home and that she would see me that night! I couldn't believe I had got to that point and it didn't feel like a big deal but I was so excited that the baby was on the way. I went home, put on the TENS, sat on my ball and had some lunch while watching Netflix but had to keep pausing it to get up on the couch to kneel and breathe through the surges. By about 2pm, I realized I needed to get back to the hospital as surges were very close together and all of a sudden there was a huge pressure and what I assume were my waters releasing. I had a little wobble at that point as I thought the baby would be born at home! It was a bit of a Hollywood movie scenario to get out the door and to the hospital in a hurry as I felt the baby was really pressing down and about to come but I listened to my tracks in the car and refocused. On admittance I was 9cm and brought straight to delivery – they initially offered me the birthing pool as I had it in my preferences but I was too far along so didn't have time. I had no admittance trace, I kept the TENS machine on throughout, the midwife and consultant were joking with me that I was still smiling (in between surges). I knelt on the bed, leaning over the top and I didn't feel the need for any other pain relief. Our baby girl was born within about 50 minutes of our arriving in the hospital at 3:50pm. Cord clamping was delayed as were all checks to allow skin-to-skin and nursing as per my preferences but I did need to have some intervention for the third stage as I was losing a little too much blood. For delivery of the placenta, I used the gas and air and I had a second-degree tear so needed a few stitches. But throughout I felt listened to and respected and that nothing was done unless it had to be. I felt empowered by the knowledge I had received from GentleBirth. Most of all I was ecstatic to welcome my daughter and when the midwife placed her under me on the bed I was the one to announce 'It's a girl!', which I will remember forever.

DOULAS

What is a Doula?

The word "doula" comes from Greece, meaning "in service." A doula is a trained professional labor assistant who understands the emotional and physical needs of a woman in labor and provides continuous support and care for the parents prenatally and throughout labor and birth. More and more hospitals are recognizing the benefits to mothers who choose to have additional birth support. A doula does not replicate the role of the midwife or nurse but complements their care. Full disclosure - I'm a little bit biased towards doulas as I'm a doula trainer for DONA International and I started Ireland's first doula service in 2005. It was my experience of having a doula with my first son Jack in 2003 that put me on the path to becoming a doula, a midwife and developing this program. Having that extra support for you and your partner whether it's at home or hospital can't be underestimated.

Along with your emotional and physical comfort, your midwife is also responsible for your clinical care and hospital protocol (charting, notes, etc.), whereas your doula is there purely for your emotional support and physical comfort measures. You have your very own cheerleader that you have personally chosen to be with you on this amazing day.

What Are the Benefits of Having a Doula?

We believe in "mothering the mother" - enabling a woman to have a much more satisfying, positive, and empowered experience before, during, and after birth, and thus allowing a baby to have a better start in life. On arrival at the hospital, you don't know the midwives and they don't know you. You will have had several visits with your doula, getting to know each other and going through your birth options. Your doula enhances your birth experience through information, support, empathy, and physical assistance.

In over 20 years of worldwide research, women supported by a doula during labor have been shown to have:

- Significant reduction in cesarean rates
- 25% shorter labor
- 60% reduction in epidural requests
- 30% reduction in analgesia use
- 40% reduction in forceps delivery

Consider this: If the benefits of doula care were available in a pill, it would be as crucial as folate in early pregnancy and unethical not to use it.

For more information, visit http://www.DONA.org.

█ MAKING INFORMED CHOICES

Every mom should be enabled to make informed choices about the care you receive during pregnancy, childbirth and afterward.

Why Is It Important? As a parent, you have the opportunity and responsibility to make many important decisions about your care during pregnancy, birth, and the time after birth. The decisions you make and the maternity care you receive can have lasting effects on the health and well- being of your baby, yourself, and your family.

It is the responsibility of professionals involved in your care to explain what your choices are, to provide clear, unbiased, and easy-to-understand information, and to support you in considering your options and making your decisions. The choices you make should be respected and supported.

It is always important to understand whether there is a good rationale for any procedure, drug, test, or treatment that is being given or offered to you. In many care settings, certain practices are used freely and even routinely, whether or not the mother or babies actually need it, but as a way of managing staffing levels, especially in a busy hospital.

Although these practices may be of value to women or babies in certain rare situations, they are usually unnecessary for most.

They can be disruptive and uncomfortable, can cause more serious side effects, and can lead to the use of other interventions. For these reasons, interventions should not be used routinely or unnecessarily, but on a case-by-case basis, not just because it is hospital policy or your caregiver's normal practice.

WHAT DOES MAKING INFORMED CHOICES MEAN?

Making informed decisions means learning and thinking about the best information available on birth options and then deciding what's right for you.

The BRAIN technique provides a framework for finding and organizing information in order to make an informed choice. This will help ensure that you can get answers to all of your questions and have access to the kind of care that is right for you. It is useful to practice the BRAIN technique, as it can be used for any daily decision making that you will need to do, not just within the context of pregnancy, birth, and postpartum. With practice, this framework will come naturally in times of stress.

WHAT CAN I DO TO HELP ENSURE THAT THE CARE THAT I RECEIVE DURING LABOR AND BIRTH WILL BE BEST FOR MY BABY?

Your choice of caregiver and choice of birth setting can have a major impact on the care that you receive during labor and birth. US research indicated that the biggest influence on whether you will have a cesarean is not your age or pregnancy complications but the hospital you choose. You may need to explore several possibilities to find a caregiver and birth setting that offer care consistent with the best evidence and with your needs and preferences. When parents find out that most routine labor procedures found in many hospitals are not based on sound evidence it's quite sobering. Like you, I assumed that everything done to my baby and me must be evidence-based... mustn't it? In a perfect world it would be but we're far from it.

It isn't possible to know ahead of time exactly what your labor experience will be like. Being as informed as possible in advance will help you deal confidently with any new decisions that may arise at the time. It is important to learn about your options, get answers to your questions, and think about your preferences well before labor begins. Be sure your partner is also aware of your wishes and is prepared to speak on your behalf if the need arises. (A doula does not speak on your behalf; her role is to help you find your voice and feel confident using it in labor if needed). The BRAIN tool is very helpful for parents but, if you are in a stressful situation, you need to do the STOP technique first so that you can access the part of your brain that will help you put the tool to good use. If the 'downstairs' brain is firing off and in a panic, it will shut down your access to the 'upstairs' brain, making it almost impossible to take in any information and make rational intentional decisions.

USE YOUR "BRAIN" TO MAKE INFORMED CHOICES

Benefits

Risks

Alternatives

Intuition

Nothing (ask for some more time)

The GentleBirth philosophy does not advocate refusing medical assistance. We encourage all parents to discuss their birth options during the prenatal period and during the birth process. Our philosophy promotes individualized care for mom and baby rather than routine (one size fits all) care for our GentleBirth families.

BIRTH STORY

First-Time Mom's Experience

Our baby arrived a few days early in Holles Street last week and he's just perfect! Birth was great too, drug-free, just used the TENS machine and that's it. My waters broke (all clear) on Friday 5th evening and we went into Holles St., they did a trace and allowed me to go home until Sunday morning 8am before they induced me. I managed to get them to extend the time allowed and high-tailed it to an acupuncturist on Saturday morning. My contractions started at 3pm later that day on Saturday 6th. We went back into Holles St around 2am on Sunday morning, and I was 2cm dilated and we stayed in the delivery suite. Midwives were great and really went with the birth plan, except for one that I had to have stern words with while trying to manage the contractions!

Hardest stage for me was definitely the pushing, but otherwise it was all manageable. My placenta came out by itself, 5 seconds after I started skin-to-skin! Couldn't believe it! It just dropped out! Honestly, the hardest part was navigating your way through their system. It's not that they're trying to be obstructive, it's just they have procedures, which I understand. I really had to have words with one midwife, who wasn't the one actually with me on the labor but another one, that wanted me to have the trace on constantly, move rooms, tried to break my fore waters, etc., etc. (They broke themselves 30 seconds later on the birthing stool!)

She even had a doctor come in to explain to me why the trace had to be on, and I again mentioned I was happy with intermittent.

Then she backed off and started telling me how well I was dilating and that it all looked very positive.

I feel back to my normal self, it's incredible how fast the body heals. I do put it down to sticking to the natural way. And baby's doing great, I'm breastfeeding, he was 2.98 kg at birth and is 3.1 kg already 4 days in!

INTERNATIONAL BEST PRACTICE SUPPORTS THE GENTLEBIRTH PHILOSOPHY

Most GentleBirth moms planning a hospital birth arrive at the hospital well into a spontaneous, progressing labor and they therefore avoid the routine interruptions of labor (see chart below). Achieving a calm, confident GentleBirth is more likely when you and your partner explore routine offerings with a curious attitude and choose the option that is most appropriate to your needs and circumstances at the time.

For Healthy Moms and Babies

Routine Procedures	International Best Practice?	Best Practice Recommendations
Restriction of food/ drink	No	Eat/drink at will
Continuous monitoring with EFM	No	Intermittent monitoring
Vaginal exams every 2 hours	No	Every 4 hours
Artificial release of waters	No	Waters release spontaneously.
Routine use of Pitocin IV to drive labor chemically	No	Caregiver to provide time and space for the woman to relax and progress. Unnecessary for healthy women unless labor stalls at 6cm for approximately 4 hours.
1-2 hour time limit on the 2nd stage of birth	No	Minimum of 3 hrs for first time moms. More with an epidural.
Coached pushing (purple pushing)	No	Mother leads - only with the urge to bear down in the position chosen by the mother. Passive descent encouraged for mothers with an epidural.
Episiotomy	No	In emergency situations only

Routine nose/mouth suctioning of a healthy baby	No	Unnecessary in healthy vigorous babies as it can cause a drop in infant heart rate. Wiping the nose/mouth is sufficient.
Immediate cord clamping	No	At least 1-2 minutes before clamping the cord. 'Wait for White"

Many US hospitals recommend having an IV cannula sited for the administration of drugs during the birth process. International best practice would not support this as routine care due to the risk of infection and discomfort for mom.

Another unnecessary and scientifically disputed procedure for your newborn is the routine administration of antibiotics to your baby's eyes to prevent neonatal ophthalmia, which is essentially conjunctivitis (pink eye) contracted during birth, if the mother has gonorrhea or chlamydia. If you believe you are not at risk of having these sexually transmitted diseases, you can decline this treatment. It can blur your baby's vision and may impact bonding as well as impacting all the good bacteria your baby is supposed to have when he's born that may take months to replace. Remember, your baby has just moved house very suddenly there are bright lights loud noises and it's a lot colder so giving drops that may irritate your baby's vision can be very stressful for him.

Bathing your baby soon after birth can affect your baby's ability to maintain his temperature and drop his blood sugars. This is the perfect time for lots of skin-to-skin.

There are no proven medical benefits to circumcision and it introduces risks to your newborn baby boy. The American Academy of Pediatrics no longer supports male circumcision.

Be sure to discuss these routine procedures with your health care provider ahead of time.

Dads/birth partners, remember the two key questions to help you determine if interrupting the natural flow of birth is really necessary due to a compelling reason (mom/baby's health) or is it simply due to time/resource restrictions or hospital policy.

As long as mom and baby are ok, ask for more time so you both enjoy a more relaxed, calm, confident, undisturbed, uninterrupted GentleBirth.

INDUCTION: PUTTING IT ALL INTO PERSPECTIVE

With induction rates continuing to climb, some GentleBirth moms will be faced with this dilemma, just for going past their guess dates. The WHO defines full term as 37 – 42 completed weeks. Labor is usually safest and easiest for mom and baby when it starts spontaneously. Thankfully, more and more hospitals are moving away from social inductions due to the risks to baby and are encouraging moms to wait until they have 41 completed weeks of pregnancy. Talk to your care provider about when they would recommend induction of labor without medical indications.

INDUCTION IS NOT GAME OVER

There may be medical circumstances that require induction and, although your plans may have changed, there's no need to resign yourself to the idea that you won't have a positive birth. Induction is a game-changer but it's definitely not game over for a positive birth. Your labor toolkit will be even more valuable now. All of your GentleBirth preparation will pay off as you get ready to meet your new baby. Is an induced birth a more challenging one? Sometimes … and it's more likely to be if you expect it to be. If induction is looking likely for you, I recommend using your Fear Release training and writing some new affirmations for yourself. Write a list of positive aspects of the induction to get you into a more positive frame of mind. With a little effort, you can keep your focus very positive especially with the positive induction training to help prime your body for a positive induction experience.

EAT YOUR DATES

While we're talking about due dates there's another kind of date to consider. New research suggests that eating dates in the last few weeks of pregnancy may reduce the likelihood of having to be induced, needing Pitocin to speed up your labor and reducing bleeding after birth. They are high in natural sugars so if you're monitoring your blood sugars be sure watch to how they impact your levels. The recommendations are 6 dates a day over the last 4 weeks of your pregnancy. I'm not a fan of the taste of dates myself but put it in a sticky toffee pudding and I'm there!

PREPARING FOR A POSITIVE INDUCTION

As full term approaches, talk often turns to the "eviction notice"... the weather is too hot... you're feeling heavy sleep is elusive... induction can sound enticing. For some moms, an unexpected complication means an abrupt end to the dream of a spontaneous labor waking up to the waters releasing during the night the excited anticipation of every sensation becoming something more. Induction does not mean "game over" if you've been planning to give birth without an epidural. Your birth preferences will, of course, need to adapt, but you can still maintain some control over what happens on the day and when, especially if you and baby are well. Whether your induction was good news or not, there's still lots you can do to have a positive birth experience for you and your baby.

NEED MORE TIME?

Induction policies differ, depending on the hospital you're attending and your caregiver. Asking for a few extra days is usually quite acceptable these days if you and baby are well. Many caregivers offer induction in the mistaken belief that all moms are fed up and want to end the pregnancy. It's a case of "if you don't ask, you don't get." If you are full term and are being induced because the "waters are low," sometimes the waters are just on the low side of normal and still within normal ranges. Ask if this is the case for you. Studies have shown that drinking extra fluids before a scan increases the amniotic fluid volume (as does water aerobics), so be sure you're well hydrated when going for a scan after your guess date.

A FEW DAYS BEFORE

Before you and your caregiver decide on a date for your induction, ask your caregiver for your Bishop's score, which is a scoring system that includes information such as how ready your cervix is for induction. The higher the score, the more likely your induction is to be straightforward, with minimal complications for you and your baby. If your score is low, you and your caregiver can consider moving your induction date to a later date, especially if you've had a healthy pregnancy. In the days before an induction, you may be offered a sweep or you can request one. This is an internal examination where the midwife/obstetrician tries to insert a finger into the opening of the cervix to separate the amniotic sac from the cervix and encourage the release of the hormones responsible for effacing and softening the cervix so it can open easily. You may have some spotting and crampiness after this procedure; if you have any concerns, call your maternity unit. In rare cases, the waters may accidentally release during this examination. Talk to your caregiver about the pros/cons of having a sweep.

Step 1 - Prostaglandins

For first-time moms, induction is often started with a pessary or gel (Cervidil) of synthetic hormones (prostaglandin) that is placed next to the cervix to soften it and hopefully kick-start the process. You may have several doses of this hormone over a couple of days, so resting and eating/staying hydrated are the orders of the day. If you have an epidural, eating is likely to be discouraged. You will have a period of continuous monitoring after the induction is begun and then hopefully left to your own devices for a few hours to mobilize. A second-time mom who has a soft ripe cervix may only need her waters released. Some caregivers use a drug called Misoprostol/Cytotec, which has been associated with some high profile cases. Be sure to discuss what medication is likely to be used for your induction. In some cases, a Foley bulb is used, which is like a small balloon that is inflated to stretch the cervix, causing it to release prostaglandins. It can be very effective and some hospitals send moms home to rest rather than being in the hospital, staring at the four walls and willing labor to start. Ask if it's an option for you.

Step 2 - Releasing the Waters

The next step in an induction is usually release of the waters around your baby in an attempt to encourage your baby to descend and apply more direct pressure to your cervix to dilate. You can ask for this step to be postponed for a few more hours if labor is starting to get established and you are coping well. The timing of the release of waters is dependent on how well the gel has worked or if you are already dilated with or without Step 1. During this procedure, your midwife will insert a plastic instrument (amnihook) and nick the bag of waters. The waters will continue to trickle and gush throughout the birth process, so bring a few pairs of underwear and maternity pads.

Step 3 – IV Pitocin/Syntocinon

This is the final step in a chemical induction; its function is to drive the uterus artificially to contract longer and more frequently. If you're currently at Step 2 you can ask for more time before moving to Step 3. Nipple stimulation (manually or with a breast pump) can increase your own body's natural oxytocin. You'll have an IV placed into your hand to administer the drugs. The drip is generally not given within six hours of the last dose of prostaglandin gel. The drip is turned up frequently to a maximum dose as long as your baby is tolerating the longer surges. With the drip comes continuous monitoring so movement can be restricted.

▌COMFORT STRATEGIES WITHOUT MEDICATION

You're Stronger Than You Think.

Consider having a doula whether you are being induced or not. Don't underestimate the benefits of extra support on the big day for you and your partner, as inductions can sometimes be longer. All mothers need continuous emotional support during labor, especially in a strange clinical environment like the hospital but most parents don't realize they won't have 1:1 continuous care from a nurse (especially in U.S. hospitals) where your nurse may be looking after more than one family.

Mental focus - Use your brain training 30 minutes before your induction starts so you are relaxed and keeping your adrenaline levels low. Use your positive induction training in the days leading up to the induction to get you in a positive frame of mind, especially if the idea of induction is less than appealing. Write your list of positive aspects of being induced to help shift your mindset. Bring along some items from home to make the space your own. Mammals nest in a space chosen by them, so you'll be making a new "nest" in your hospital. Items to consider include a special photo that brings back positive memories and music that transports you to a happy time in your life. These are simple ways to increase your natural pain-relieving hormones.

Slow breathing - Slow comfortable breathing is a simple way to maintain focus and feelings of control. Breathe all the way down to your baby slowly and deeply to keep you and your baby well oxygenated and relaxed.

TENS Machine - Start using your TENS machine 30 minutes before the start of your induction to give your natural pain-relieving endorphins a boost. Bring your own birth ball and use it when you're on the monitor to keep you comfortable. You can also stand or sit in a chair when staff members need to listen in to your baby. Lying flat on your back on the bed can make the sensations more intense and makes it harder for your baby to descend.

For Step 1 and Step 2, use the bath/shower; deep warm water immersion is very effective in releasing your body's own birth hormones and it can keep you more comfortable.

Acupressure techniques can be very effective during an induction.

Use your VR headset to reduce the intensity of the surges.

COMFORT STRATEGIES WITH MEDICATION

"At the end of the day after 60 hours of labor GentleBirth gave me a sense of calm and togetherness to tell people what I needed which thankfully included the epidural."
–Laura Mitchell–

Nitrous oxide is becoming more widely available throughout the U.S. and can provide excellent analgesia. It is administered through a mouthpiece as mom breathes in the "laughing gas." If mom doesn't like using it, she can stop and it is out of your system very quickly with minimal side effects for your baby.

Narcotics such as Fentanyl, Morphine or Pethidine make some moms feel quite "spaced out," sleepy, and sometimes nauseous. It passes to your baby and some babies may need help remembering to breathe when they are born. If this happens, your baby will be given a drug to reverse the side effects. It can also affect your baby's ability to breastfeed.

Epidural - Some caregivers recommend the epidural for Step 3 (Pitocin IV), as some moms find the intensity of the artificially driven surges along with tiredness more difficult to cope with. Limited mobility can make the experience more difficult. Ask for monitoring while sitting on the ball or standing if you don't have the epidural. Not all moms find the chemical surges more difficult to cope with. Keep an open mind rather than automatically having an epidural and potentially adding more complications to your baby's birth. Some of the trade-offs include an increase in instrumental births, longer labor, and an increase in temperature for mom. Only you know how well you are coping. You may surprise yourself; you're stronger than you think.

Induction can be a very positive experience and, although there are some things you have no control over during birth, you always have control over how you respond to what's happening in your experience. Be engaged and curious about your care; ask questions and talk to other GentleBirth moms who have had positive inductions.

The Bishop's score is a somewhat subjective scoring system used to determine how successful an induction of labor might be for you. The higher the score, the better. To ensure your own induction's success rate, ask about your Bishop's score. Induction with a low

Bishop's score can mean a more challenging birth for you and your baby.

BIRTH PARTNERS – TIME TO ADOPT A CURIOUS ATTITUDE

Birth partners/dads, it's important to keep the atmosphere as calm and relaxed as possible during birth, and labor is certainly no time to be debating hospital policy. A pleasant curious attitude with a smile will go a long way. If an intervention such as speeding up labor or releasing the waters is being offered, there are a few key questions that you can ask to make sure the procedure really is necessary and not just a routine procedure to rush your partner through labor. It's easy to feel intimidated by medical staff (though this is rarely intentional by the staff) and not feel confident enough to ask questions because you have no medical training, but here are a few questions to help you "protect the space" so mom can stay focused on giving birth in her own time on her own terms and cocooned in the "zone."

> Is my partner OK?
>
> Is our baby OK?

Put simply, if you don't ask for the birth you want you'll get the birth you're given.

UNEXPECTED CHANGES TO YOUR PREFERRED BIRTH PLAN (INDUCTION OR CESAREAN)

This is a powerful technique, based on CBT (cognitive behavioral therapy), to help shift your perspective from the negative to a more positive mindset in the event you develop a complication in pregnancy that changes your birth preferences significantly. Most moms have healthy normal pregnancies but, if you find yourself in this situation, you can reframe how you feel about the changes so you stay on track for a positive birth experience no matter what cards you are dealt.

We start off with the "minus" column below and define the problem. Then you move across to the plus column and find a positive; see the first example, adapted from the novel Robinson Crusoe by Daniel Defoe. The positive side always starts with BUT - as it reduces the emotional "punch" of the first sentence.

Negative	Positive Reframe
EXAMPLE - I've been shipwrecked on a remote island.	BUT I survived when everyone else drowned.
I'm being induced tomorrow due to a serious complication. This really isn't what I wanted.	BUT at least I know my baby will be in my arms very soon. BUT I'm so grateful that my midwife detected the problem so early.
My baby is transverse and I have to have a cesarean. I'm so disappointed.	BUT this is the safest way for my baby to be born. BUT I can prepare myself now and don't have the unpredictability of labor.
My blood pressure is dangerously high and I need to have an epidural to bring it down. I really wanted a natural birth.	BUT the epidural is helping me have the safest birth for my baby. BUT I don't need it for pain relief; I'm coping with the sensations really well.
My iron levels might be too low to safely have my homebirth.	BUT I am now increasing my iron for the safest birth for my baby and me.

Whatever cards you've been dealt that have derailed your plans for your GentleBirth, do the exercise above, and then write down five positives about this new birth plan.

GOLDILOCKS AND THE THREE PERFECTLY SIZED BABIES

Remember the bedtime story of Goldilocks? Goldilocks tried the three chairs ... one was too big... one was too small and one was just right...... what is the 'just right' sized baby?

Several times a month I'm contacted by moms who have had a recent ultrasound and have been told that their baby is measuring too big or too small, so I thought this issue needed addressing from an evidence standpoint as a midwife and as a mom who gave birth to a 10lb 7oz baby boy at home with a midwife, doula and just a slight perineal graze.

Going for a scan is generally an exciting time, as you get to take a peek at your baby in his little world. But in the back of every mom's mind is the worry that something unexpected may show up on the scan. You're caught between watching the strange shapes on the screen and watching the sonographer's facial expressions looking for clues that something's not quite right. You probably even forget to breathe if you have a particularly quiet sonographer as she clicks and concentrates.

WHAT'S THE BIG DEAL ABOUT BIG BABIES?

I've found that although there is an international definition for 'big' babies sometimes the prediction of a 'big' baby is in the eye of the beholder (your OB) if you're not particularly tall. The research suggests that a baby is considered to be big when it weighs more than 4,000 grams (8 pounds 13 ounces) at birth, and others say a baby is big if it weighs more than 4,500 grams (9 pounds, 15 ounces).

Big babies are more likely to experience problems with their shoulders being born (shoulder dystocia), but around half of all babies who have this problem are of 'normal' weight. Epidurals and instrumental births add to this problem. Babies need lots of room to maneuver through the pelvis and, if your pelvis is closed (i.e., you're flat on your back), it makes it harder for baby. An 'open' pelvis is an upright pelvis or at least side lying. Instrumental births are a risk factor for shoulder dystocia in all babies - big or small. Shoulder dystocia is a medical emergency but, in most cases, it can be resolved by changing mom's position to facilitate opening the pelvis more.

A 2009 study reported that your caregiver's suspicion of a big baby is, in fact, more dangerous than the baby itself! Moms who were suspected of having a big baby (and actually ended up having one) had three times the induction rate, more than triple the C-section rate, and a quadrupling of complications for mom compared to women whose obstetricians didn't think their baby was big and who ended up having a surprise big baby in the end. Scans are notoriously inaccurate, especially late in your pregnancy.

Inductions come along with a long list of potential problems for you and your baby and there is no evidence to support inducing early to 'stop baby getting any bigger.' Induction increases the likelihood of complications instead of reducing them.

I can only imagine how stressful it can be to be told your baby is measuring large at 35 weeks knowing you have potentially another 5+ weeks to go. Especially when this discussion is not happening within the context of how the pelvis shifts and moves in labor and how your baby's head is made up of flexible plates that overlap as baby descends. As your baby grows in those next five weeks, he's laying down fat reserves on his back, not his head! I was expecting a bigger baby this time around as Jack was 8lbs 15oz but never dreamed Cooper would be over 10lbs (and I was not diabetic). Babies born to moms with uncontrolled diabetes tend to be on the larger size due to the extra sugar in mom's bloodstream. If your diabetes is well controlled and your sugars have been stable, this is not something for you to be worried about. I'm quite sure the last few weeks of my pregnancy would have been very different if I'd had a late scan and no doubt the worry would have impacted my labor, which would probably have become a self-fulfilling prophecy.

▌PARENTS SPEAK

"My son, first baby, was exactly 9lbs when born. In all scans, he had been measuring on the bigger side but no one had made any comments until, at 38 weeks, one midwife asked me what I was eating, as the baby was big! I was devastated as I thought it was all my fault and I wouldn't be able to have a home birth with the community midwives. A week later, a different midwife had a feel and she said I was grand and the baby wasn't that big. Anyway, I delivered my 9lb baby with just gas and air, turns out he was long not fat and, seeing as his dad is 6ft 4, I wasn't surprised. He continued to grow grow grow and was off the charts at his last developmental check. He is 1 and wears 2-year-old clothes. So my baby was the perfect size for my body, yes it stung pushing him out but I was absolutely fine after and don't think a smaller baby would have felt much different." – Aoife

"The whole way through my pregnancy, I had been measuring average no one even mentioned the words "big baby"! But Katie was born 9lb 9oz! I got through it with just gas and air and TENS machine but have to say the midwife was brilliant too, advising to pause when baby's head was emerging and, with that advice, baby was born with only slight grazing!" – Amanda

▌IS SMALLER BETTER?

We know that scans are rarely accurate and that goes for predicting small but healthy babies, too. As a precaution, we're always going to monitor your baby's weight gain and blood flow through the placenta more thoroughly if we think your baby's growth has slowed down significantly. We'll also consider your lifestyle (smoking/stress) and your diet. A sick baby is definitely better off on the outside receiving medical care than on the inside if he's not growing. Up until recently, it was thought that a baby that was in the 10th percentile of growth (meaning 90% of other babies are likely to be larger) needed to be born but new international guidelines suggest that most of these babies are perfectly healthy but they're just small. Chances are mom has had small healthy babies in the past or, if this is her first, when we look at the parents we can see that they are usually small framed themselves and were probably smaller babies at birth too. Only the babies that fall into the 3rd percentile (if all else is well) require additional monitoring and perhaps an early birth. For more information ask your careprovider about the PORTO study.

THINGS YOU CAN DO

Big or small - all babies do better when mom has a healthy balanced diet, is getting some exercise, reducing stress, increasing joy and avoiding cigarettes/ drugs.

Talk to your caregiver about the evidence against induction/ cesarean for suspected big or small babies based on international best practice.

BREECH BABY

I had an opportunity to work with a first time mom with a baby who was unexpectedly breech (butt first instead of head first). She was a few days shy of being full term and her waters released. The usual practice in this particular hospital is to have a cesarean but as mom wasn't showing any signs of labor and it was a busy day she was admitted and left to her own devices for the day. She put on the App, rested and adjusted to the new plan ahead with her partner– as she was really hoping for a water birth. Mom had been very anxious in early pregnancy and although disappointed now she was excited to meet her baby. That evening Mom began to complain about some lower backache... and knowing how GentleBirth moms can be 'sneaky' birthers (not feeling much discomfort) I asked her to time the sensations to see if there was any pattern to this backache. I went to get her a heat pack for her lower back and sure enough these sensations were starting to come every 10 minutes. I mentioned it to some of the senior midwives that we needed to keep an eye on this mom but when they looked in on her mom was dozing with headphones on and not a bother on her. In fact I was reprimanded for suggesting mom was in labor... but when you've seen enough GentleBirths you pick up on the very subtle signs of labor progress without a mom screaming the hospital down. About an hour later this pattern of sensations was beginning to feel more like period pain. Here's the thing – theater staff don't like surprises (and who can blame them in their line of work) so they would really like a heads up if a mom who is going to be having a cesarean starts to labor). I asked a senior midwife to come and check on this mom... and sure enough mom was found to be 10cm. Mom was delighted! She had a natural labor with only a heat pack and very little pain – theater staff were not so delighted with this unexpected patient. I ended up having an inquisition the next day about what magic was in GentleBirth to 'make' the mother labor so quickly – especially as her baby was breech. I explained that it was not magic – just the reduction of fear which makes labor harder and more painful. They weren't convinced – imagine if it were true and nobody needed Pitocin anymore – just pop on your GentleBirth and pop out your baby!

WHEN IS BREECH POSITION CONSIDERED A PROBLEM?

More and more I'm reading reports of worried moms leaving scans as early as 28 weeks having been informed that their baby is breech.

Moms then spend the next several weeks stressed, anxious and doing strange things with frozen bags of peas and flashlights in an attempt to coax their baby into a head down position and avoid a cesarean. Before 36 weeks your baby has plenty of room to flip into multiple positions several times a day (and probably once or twice before dawn too).

First things first - less than 5% of babies stay breech (butt first) at full term so you have plenty of time and still have options to consider.

Let's slow that roll a little as the position of your baby is really of no importance until you reach 35-36 weeks...then your midwife/doctor will start to focus a little more on the 'plan' if your baby stays in a breech position.

ECV – ask if there's a breech clinic in your hospital if you haven't already been referred for an External Cephalic Version – this is an external manipulation of your baby to nudge him into a head down position – the success rate is about 50% but it's definitely worth a try before agreeing to major abdominal surgery (cesarean birth). ECV is an option for most healthy mums with no complications including women who have had a previous cesarean birth. An ECV is not a gentle massage but quite firm and can be quite uncomfortable (but it's usually over quickly) and if your consultant feels too much resistance they won't continue. If you find it very painful you can always ask to stop.

Complimentary therapies include acupuncture (or moxa), hypnosis (deeply relaxing and oxygenating the uterine muscles gives baby more room) and Spinning Babies. There is a Breech Baby Turn hypnosis session in the GentleBirth App that Moms have great success with. I recommend moms use it for 10 days and do acupuncture sessions also. In one research paper on the use of hypnosis 80% of babies turned and stayed head down. There is also the Webster Technique facilitated by a Chiropractor. But other than hypnosis and acupuncture there are very few good studies on the effectiveness of these therapies.

Although less common breech vaginal birth can be a safe option as long as the care provider is skilled in breech birth. The type of breech will also determine if a vaginal birth is a safe option (Frank breech is considered the safest). For a first time mom you may have to do a little research to find a consultant willing to support a vaginal breech birth. It's important to weigh up the pros/cons of a vaginal breech birth and a planned cesarean birth – both carry risks for mom and baby. New research suggests a breech birth without an epidural is beneficial for mum and baby as mum can move into positions that encourage her baby to move through the pelvis more easily. If a breech birth is something you're considering check out the revolutionary work of German obstetrician Frank Louwen.

If you've tried everything and a cesarean birth looks likely you can make that experience as positive as possible.

- Ask to wait until you have the first sign of labor – then you know your baby is ready to be born and is less likely to have breathing difficulties.
- Plan your cesarean date at 40 weeks or later so your baby gets those extra few days for development and who knows your baby might still turn at the last minute especially if this isn't your first baby.
- Read up about seeding your baby's gut so your baby is exposed to similar 'friendly' bacteria he would have been colonized with if he had been born vaginally.
- Write birth preferences that include immediate skin to skin in theater and recovery room and delayed cord clamping so your baby's birth can be as gentle and positive as possible.

▌BACTERIA CAN BE GOOD FOR YOUR BABY

Most people think of bacteria as germs that make you sick but, in fact, they are also critical to keeping you healthy. Scientists now think of the microbiome as an organ and it weighs about the same as your brain.

In pregnancy the level of bacteria changes in the vagina and digestive system.

- Changes in gut mean mom's body is better at taking nutrients from food.
- Low Ph makes vagina more acidic to reduce bacteria ascending to the uterus.
- Lactobacillus bacteria also have inbuilt antibiotics to kill dangerous bacteria.
- These first microbes train your baby's immune system.
- Untreated depression changes your microbes.

Recently there was a media storm over a study that suggested children born by cesarean were more likely to become obese. It's not clear why this is the case and many of the reports surrounding this study left out an important detail that could hold the key – gut bacteria. A small study published in *Nature* a year previously suggested a distinct link between the composition of our gut microbiota and incidence of obesity and related metabolic conditions, including cardiovascular disorders and diabetes.

▌WHAT IS GUT BACTERIA – ▌AND WHY DO WE NEED IT?

- Your body contains trillions of cells, and many of these microorganisms do a great job training our immune system by recognizing disease-producing bacteria, producing Vitamin K. These special microorganisms are essential for health and wellbeing, but what if being born via cesarean means your baby has missed out on what could be considered his first immunization? A baby is exposed to mom's feces as he's being born vaginally (bifidobacteria) – this is a lactic acid bacteria that boosts baby's energy after birth. It breaks down the sugars in breast milk and coats your baby's intestine and inhibits the growth of disease-causing bacteria. These smart microbes create their own antibiotics to kick out any pathogenic (bad) bacteria. Antibiotics alter your baby's microbiome for up to 12 months, especially if not breastfed. The good news is that breastfeeding modifies some of the effects of a cesarean birth – it's like an insurance policy, especially if you had a cesarean and/or antibiotics in labor.

The types of bacteria in the guts of babies born by cesarean tend to differ from those born vaginally. Babies born vaginally are colonized by lactobacillus, whereas babies born by cesarean have more pathogenic (disease-causing) bacteria such as staphylococcus. Interestingly, a recent study has shown that mice could be made obese or lean just by changing their gut bacteria. When a baby is born vaginally, he is exposed to your vaginal and intestinal flora, which is the start of your baby's colonization (also known as seeding). In a planned cesarean, this doesn't happen and babies can end up being colonized with more disease-causing bacteria instead of 'friendly' bacteria. Some studies are showing a difference in these microorganisms even seven years later between babies born vaginally and babies born by cesarean (breastfeeding helps!)

WHAT DOES THIS MEAN FOR YOUR BABY?

This area of research is exploding and we still have a lot to learn. It seems that vaginal birth 'switches on' your baby's immunity, and certain genes. Some studies are suggesting an increased risk for allergies in cesarean-born babies. If not breastfed, your baby is also missing out on the benefits of breastfeeding, which also protects the baby's gut. Studies also show that between 64 and 82 percent of reported cases of MRSA skin infections in newborns occurred in infants born by cesarean. Your baby's immune system is suppressed at birth to 'trick' your body to not reject the pregnancy (it lasts about 3 weeks after birth so microbes can colonize the gut). But what if the first microbes are from other people or equipment in theater? Scientists believe that if your baby's immune system isn't trained properly it can't recognize what the good/bad bacteria are.

Cesareans have also been associated with a significantly increased rate of asthma, especially in girls, and allergic rhinitis. This increase was even more apparent looking at the risk of asthma which was increased by 60 percent in baby girls who underwent a repeat cesarean without ruptured membranes (waters breaking), versus those babies with waters released and/or labor prior to the cesarean. Type 1 diabetes has been on the increase, and studies have found a 19 percent increase in Type 1 diabetes in cesarean children. So labor seems to have protective factors for babies, or at minimum a cesarean after the waters have been released.

But, as we learn more about these microorganisms and their role in our health, more questions need answering. How do antibiotics during pregnancy, labor, or right before a cesarean impact the colonization of your baby's gut with this 'friendly' bacteria? How our babies are born may have far-reaching consequences that we are just starting to understand. This becomes even more important as cesarean rates increase and the lack of meaningful support by healthcare professionals for VBAC.

HOW CAN YOU HELP YOUR BABY GET MORE 'FRIENDLY' BACTERIA AFTER BIRTH?

There's no doubt that cesareans are necessary and save lives, but what if you could actively help reduce your baby's risk of allergic reactions and potential health problems by 'seeding' your baby's gut with all the good bacteria?

There are growing reports of moms and midwives promoting the use of vaginal swabs pre-cesarean which is then wiped over baby after the baby is born. So your baby gets your bacteria and not the bacteria from the hospital wall! A milliliter of vaginal fluid contains, on average, around 100 million microorganisms from 5-10 species, 95 percent of which are from the lactobacillus family (the good stuff!).

This is an emerging area of research and there is limited available evidence to support this practice, but it does seem to make sense. Other ways to seed your baby include establishing breastfeeding after your cesarean and maybe probiotic supplements. Some midwives in the US are taking a 'bottom' up approach and attempting to seed the baby by using natural live yogurt as a nappy cream in the first days following a cesarean. These good bacteria seem to tolerate life outside of the body, so it's likely that your baby can reap the benefits of this odd but inventive practice.

However, the ideal bacteria for baby to receive are of course yours. Some women having planned cesareans are proactively taking samples of their vaginal secretions (with their finger) before going to the theater and placing the fluid around their nipples so their baby is exposed to that good bacteria as soon as possible.

At worst you might feel a bit weird doing this (nobody has to know) – at best you may reduce your baby's risk of health problems in later life. Some experts feel this puts babies at risk of contracting GBS or other infections but, if the cesarean hadn't happened, the baby would have been exposed to those bacteria anyway.

Microbiome research is in its infancy and, as it is evolving, there has been some debate on whether vaginal 'seeding' is safe for a baby born to a mom who is GBS+. Talk to your care provider if you are considering this option.

Microbiome influences pain and behavior such as anxiety.

▌GBAC - GENTLEBIRTH AFTER CESAREAN

If you've previously had a cesarean and are planning a vaginal birth, there are a couple of things to consider to make this next experience more empowering and positive.

Depending on where you are giving birth, you may find there is resistance to VBAC or that there will be strict time limits on how long your birth process will last or how long "over" your EDD you can go before there is pressure to do something. Although much talked about, it's actually quite rare for your previous scar to open in a spontaneous birth and, in the unlikely event that it does happen, it is rarely fatal for mom or her baby.

One of the keys to a successful VBAC is a supportive caregiver; it's better to find out in the early stages of your pregnancy that you've hired the right (or wrong) person for the job rather than to find out at 38 weeks that your caregiver may talk the talk but doesn't walk the walk when it comes to VBAC. For many VBAC moms, their confidence in their body's ability has been severely knocked and will take time to rebuild. Daily conditioning with your GentleBirth VBAC brain training is critical to restoring your faith in birth. Around 70% of moms who choose VBAC go on to have straightforward births. Write some affirmations for yourself around any specific fears you have for your VBAC.

Let's face it, VBAC spells FEAR to many obstetricians, to the media, to your family, and very often to you yourself. These fears are compounded by the use of negative priming vocabulary, such as "trial of labor" "scar," "rupture," "failure to progress," "distress" … do any of these words bring up images of calm, confident, gentle birthing? No. The use of these words reinforces the belief that our bodies are broken and reaffirms in our subconscious mind that birth is an accident waiting to happen.

Having a VBAC can be hard work (psychologically) - finding the right caregiver, gaining support from your birth partner, trusting yourself. If you had a very traumatic birth experience the first time around, then it's very likely that your subconscious mind believes that birth is to be feared and will work hard to create that reality.

After a cesarean birth, there can be a huge cloud of distrust that surrounds the new mom... distrust of her body... distrust of the medical profession, sometimes distrust of the doctor she believed would "do no harm" or of routine policies that may have contributed to having a surgical birth. I've had the wonderful pleasure of watching this cloud slowly disappear with GentleBirth couples and see it replaced with renewed confidence, faith, and even excitement for the birth process to begin. For more information on VBAC, visit http://www. VBACFacts.com or contact ICAN (International Cesarean Awareness Network) or find a GentleBirth VBAC class in your community.

▌AFFIRMATIONS FOR VBAC

- I can do it!
- My body rocks!
- My surges are gentle but strong.
- VBAC is a healthy and safe choice.
- I am ready for whatever comes my way on the day.
- I can handle whatever type of birth I am given. My baby and I are doing this together.
- I know what's best for my baby. I trust my body. My confidence is growing every day.
- I am ready.
- I want this.
- Yes!
- My body is strong.

- I choose healthy options to prepare my body and mind for birth. My baby knows how to be born.
- All is well.

BIRTH STORY

Wonderful VBAC Birth

So on the morning of Tuesday 30th April I woke at 1 am needing to pee. Got back into bed and felt a surge at 1:09am, didn't think much of it and snuggled back down to sleep. By 1:50am I was having strong surges every 5/6 minutes and couldn't sleep through them, so decided to text Mary (our doula) and have a cup of tea. I just knew that this was finally it, our baby was coming to meet us at long last! I texted my friend Tania, who was going to keep some close friends informed of the goings-on. Twenty minutes later the surges were every 4/5 minutes and I hadn't heard back from Mary so I rang her as it would take her an hour to get to our house. I had a few contractions while on the phone and she knew by the fact I couldn't talk through them things were definitely happening. My friend Tania said she would stay up and keep me company by text until Mary arrived as I was letting hubbie sleep on. I lit some incense and candles and knew that I didn't want the TV or laptop on, so started some crochet. I didn't get much of it done as kept having to re-do it, but it helped me focus. I got hubbie up then to put on the TENS machine as things were pretty intense and now every 3/4 minutes. Just before Mary arrived, I asked hubbie to get up to ring CUMH and his mom to let them know we'd need to go soon. I knew if I waited much longer I wouldn't be able for the car journey. When the surges were happening, all I could do was breathe through them and tune everything out. I just kept repeating in my head "I can do anything for a minute." Mary arrived and then Graham's mom so we decided to go straight to CUMH. The pressure in the car was very intense and I hated being stuck in the one position. We got to CUMH at about 4:30am and went to the waiting room. They weren't massively busy but all staff occupied so we were in the waiting room for about 90 minutes, luckily just the three of us because, at this stage during the surges, I was kneeling on all fours on the floor and moaning. Mary plugged in her electric oil burner with a relaxing blend and was using counter pressure on my hips during the contractions, which were every 2-3 minutes and it was such a help. By 5:30am, I watched the sun start to rise and felt it was a beautiful day to birth a baby! But the TENS was starting to annoy the f*ck out of me and I knew I needed some gas and air to help me through the surges. Finally got into triage at 6am and examined to be told was "just about 3-4cm dilated." I hated that midwife right then as it was what I was told on being admitted in labor with Charlotte. She wanted me on the CTG then and told me I would have to lie or stand, squatting on the floor was not an option. I hated her even more then as I knew there was no way I could lie on that bed for 20 minutes. Anyway, I said I'd stand, she put on the trace and Graham came in to me, he helped support me upright during the surges and reassured me I was doing an amazing job. We overheard the midwife ring through to labor ward and neither of us were too impressed with what we heard or her attitude when she came back into us but we chose to ignore her as, once we got to delivery, we wouldn't have to see her again. So after the trace we were waiting another while to go down as there was rooms free but no staff. I think we got downstairs at about 7am. Midwife we got was nice but said no to pool as it was against VBAC protocol as I would need continuous trace. I said I would agree to this as long as it didn't stop me moving about as no way I could be lying in bed constantly. I knew that if that happened it would be end of my VBAC. She was supportive of this and got me a gym ball so I was on that with the Entonox on the trace and managing well. 8am and staff changeover happened. We got a midwife called Catherine, (which was the name we had agreed as a middle name if we had a girl as it's my sister's middle name) and a student midwife called Vicky (my middle name is Victoria). I took this as a sign these ladies were going to help me have my VBAC! Just after the changeover, the ob and her team came in. The cons was a b*tch. I hated her and she didn't like me much either as she wanted to have me examined sooner rather than later and if no progression wanted to rupture my waters. I straight out told her no and she then started to spout about uterine rupture, told her I knew the risks and how low the percentage was. Said again breaking of waters was not happening, to which she replied "So you're willing to risk your uterus rupturing as opposed to having your waters broken?" Yes, says I! She made the other doc note on my chart I'd been informed blah blah blah. The last doc out was the doc who had seen me in A&E last week when I had the bleeding and, as she left, said "good luck" and gave me a big smile. Then had a good laugh with Catherine, Vicky, and Mary about how I'd told the cons what's what and took no shit. I wanted the loo so Catherine took me off the trace. I sat on the loo for a while, but then decided to chance asking Catherine could I have a bath, as she seemed really supportive of our birth preferences and a hands-off approach from her. She ran the bath and we sneaked over as doc had said explicitly no to pool and bath due to continuous trace, blah blah. In the bath for a while, sucking on Entonox, moaning through the surges but felt I was starting to panic a bit and needed something more. Really didn't want Pethidine as felt this was where my labor had slowed the last time and DEF didn't want the epidural. So I chatted with Graham, Mary, and Catherine about options. Decided Catherine would do exam and then we'd form a plan. I was terrified of another exam and being told "only 4cm" I was so afraid I wouldn't get past the point things stalled on Charlotte. Such a relief when Catherine said I was "a loose 8cm." I seriously cannot explain how elated I felt, that my body had done this and knew that there was no way this was going to be a section! I was getting my VBAC. So my waters were bulging A LOT and Catherine said that was what was contributing to the amount of pressure down below. My options were for her to release them to relieve some of the pressure or for me to have Pethidine to take the edge off things and wait for them to release themselves. I felt strongly I wanted my membranes to release themselves and at this point felt Pethidine wouldn't slow things down, so opted for that. Think that was about 10am. Timings are a bit off in my head. So after that I was on the ball again, then on the toilet for a while but I couldn't settle and decided the shower might be nice. Hopped in with the hot spray directed onto my lower back, Entonox in my mouth, and was there for a while. Pethidine definitely took the edge off but was feeling serious pressure between my legs, reached down and could feel something, but knew waters still intact so said I thought Catherine should check me again. She did and said that there was a big cervical lip and if she pushed it back I was 10cm, but it was slipping back over baby's head. She said she felt it was preventing waters releasing themselves. So we agreed she'd break them. The relief from that was unreal!! That was at about 11am, I think. Catherine then wanted to do a CTG, I only found out after Alicia was born it was because there was meconium in the waters. I was on the gym ball and poor Vicky was having to hold the CTG in place the whole time.

So after a while I was unsettled again and got on the bed, kneeling over the back of it. I felt major pressure and asked Catherine to check me as I could feel something between my legs. She checked and told me we'd hit double digits! I was so pleased with myself and knew we'd soon meet our beautiful baby. So I was standing beside the bed when I felt Alicia start to descend. I stayed in this position for a while with legs spread and could feel her slowly making her way further down with each surge. It was surreal and amazing. But I wouldn't settle so got into the kneeling on the bed again. Graham was standing beside me holding my hand and telling me how fab I was doing, Mary was behind me taking pictures as our daughter's head emerged. A couple more surges and some intense pressure and our daughter slid out onto the bed between my legs in a gush of fluids. She let out a big roar of indignation and I reached down and lifted her up to my chest. I saw we had another girl and looked over to Graham to tell him. He was crying and shaking and I have never loved him so much. I announced to everyone we had another beautiful girl and turned to sit with her in my arms. Within about 15 minutes Alicia started to nurse all by herself pretty much. We wanted delayed cord clamping so really at this point it was waiting for the cord to stop pulsing. I'm not sure how long this took, but think it was about 30 minutes, the cord was completely white when Graham cut it. Then he had cuddles with Alicia while Catherine cleaned me up and she said I'd need a stitch due to second-degree tear. We rang family and texted close friends to inform them Alicia was here. Vicky got us all tea and toast, which was amazing! Even though I'd had smoothies and snacks during the whole labor I was starving!! Mary left a bit after that and then Catherine went on her lunch break so we were left just the three of us until about 4/4:30pm, when we transferred upstairs.

2ND VBAC

Our third daughter arrived this morning - five hours of moderate surges, just getting ready to head to the hospital after three intense ones when waters went in the bathroom and 23 minutes/5 surges later, I was sat on the floor holding Matilda! Paramedics arrived ten minutes later and took us in to be checked. Long but shallow tear so I have some stitches, but otherwise all well with us both not quite as gentle as I'd have imagined at the end but only for GB (and our wonderful doula, Mary Tighe). I'm not sure DH and I would have coped the way we had to!

> GentleBirth VBAC Mom
>
> "Empowering, instinctive, natural, absolutely wonderful! I felt really connected to my body, my baby, my husband, the midwives and consultant right throughout labor and birth. We worked as a complete partnership."

BABY, BREASTFEEDING AND BEYOND

Mothers don't breastfeed, babies breastfeed.
Babies know how if we let them"
–Nils Bergman–

▌BREASTFEEDING AND YOUR BRAIN

Most GentleBirth moms breastfeed (96%) but not all of them start off feeling confident in their abilities. In the same way you've been practicing the thought that childbirth has to be long, difficult, and horribly painful, a lot of moms have learned that breastfeeding is also fraught with pain and must be hard work to get established. (More 'dodgy' wiring in the brain that needs to be rewired). Yet other mammals don't seem to have these problems have you ever heard of a cat complaining of sore nipples and our feline friends probably have four or five hungry mouths to feed - at one time! All newborn mammals know how to find their food source: They are born with highly sensitive built-in instincts to crawl to the breast and feed with little help from mom. If your expectations of breastfeeding aren't very positive at the moment, you can start off by writing out some affirmations for yourself around breastfeeding. This is where your meditation practice will really pay off, you have been learning to catch that negative voice whispering to you that you can't successfully breastfeed – catch the thought, challenge the thought and change it.

▌PREPARING FOR BREASTFEEDING SUCCESS

In not so recent times mothers used to be advised to scrub their nipples in the shower to 'toughen them up' in preparation for breastfeeding. Thankfully that kind of 'preparation' is no longer advised as it can damage your nipples as well as being torture when your nipples are already sensitive due to pregnancy hormones. When your baby is latched properly breastfeeding isn't painful. Although breastfeeding is instinctual for babies - all mammals know where and how to get their food source to survive - we have made things difficult for ourselves so here are a few tips to help you prepare for a positive breastfeeding journey.

You may be living in a country where breastfeeding rates are low. It's not because your breasts are different from those in Norway, where more than 95% of women breastfeed. The problem has a lot more to do with our brains than our boobs – your mindset and expectations about breastfeeding.

- Staff members don't always have time to spend with breastfeeding mothers and, if this is your first baby and the hospital is busy, support may be minimal.
- Babies are not born hungry – they're born 'skin hungry.'

- Your newborn baby's tummy is about the size of a cherry; all it can take is about a teaspoon of colostrum on that first day or so.
- Get along to a breastfeeding support group before your baby arrives (go tomorrow).
- Find a breastfeeding 'buddy' for around your EDD so you have informational support on hand immediately.
- Take a breastfeeding class - with your partner. If your hospital doesn't encourage partners, then take a private breastfeeding class.
- The 2nd night can be hard when your newborn wants lots of skin-to-skin and seems to feed all the time - this is totally normal (he'll do it around day 10 too, when your baby has a growth spurt).
- Hire a postpartum doula to come and look after you for a few hours the first week you are home and to help you with breastfeeding.
- Breastfeeding should not be painful (it may feel a bit strange at first) - if it is, ask for help early and often. Consider getting a Lactation consultant for a visit the day you get home.
- Watch lots of online videos on biological nurturing or 'laid-back breastfeeding'. Forget trying all the contortionist breastfeeding 'holds' for the first week.
- Stay in bed for the first week until you and baby get the hang of things - restrict visitors. I know this is not easy if you have a toddler already at home, which is all the more reason to enlist the help of friends, family, or a postpartum doula.
- If it's painful - get help immediately.
- If it's painful - get help immediately (seeing a theme?)

A couple of great books to read in pregnancy are *Breastfeeding Made Simple* by Nancy Morbacher and *Sweet Sleep* - La Leche League and *The Womanly Art of Breastfeeding* by La Leche League.

THE BREASTFEEDING MINDSET

Why is breastfeeding so easy for some mothers, while for others it seems like torture? Many factors come into play: self-confidence, childhood experiences (including parental role modeling), motivation, cultural norms, body image, as well as beliefs and expectations about the potential health benefits and perceived unpleasant aspects of breastfeeding. All of these help shape our attitudes (conscious or unconscious).

Mindset influences behavior and breastfeeding success doesn't start with that first latch. It begins months before your baby arrives. I've found that most breastfeeding problems have little to do with your breast or your baby – but what's happening in your brain.

To truly be ready to successfully breastfeed, you need to cultivate a mindset that goes far beyond just having the techniques and latch (and all of those 'pretzel-like' positions that should be reserved for a Cirque du Soleil performance). You can learn those in any breastfeeding class. But as you've been learning throughout this book, the key to success in any stressful situation (breastfeeding can be intense and stressful in the very beginning) - is your ability to manage your thoughts, your anxiety, and your fears. Your ability to observe your mind and the negative stories it's likely telling you is paramount to your ability to thrive in the first few weeks of breastfeeding.

A fixed negative mindset believes that breastfeeding is too difficult, embarrassing, painful, exhausting, or too time-consuming. If you have a positive breastfeeding mindset, you're likely to think that breastfeeding is not only good for you, it's good for the baby, too, it gives you lots of bonding time with your baby....and makes you feel really good.

As well as a good breastfeeding class that will show you laid-back breastfeeding (biological nurturing) positions, you'll also need the following head edge for a more positive and enjoyable breastfeeding journey;

1. WTF
   Where's the focus? Shifting your focus to what's going right instead of what's going wrong is one of the most important skills to master and also one of the hardest. Practicing gratitude helps us to find the good more frequently.

2. Mindful Compassion. When the 'storytelling' mind has free range in your head, it's like kryptonite to breastfeeding success. When you're tired and sore it's easy to focus on the negatives which can leave you feeling overwhelmed and ready to pack it in. Practicing mindfulness lets you become more aware of the negativity bias so you can catch it when your mind starts slipping over to the 'dark' side.

3. Mental Toughness
   The first week with a newborn may be the most challenging week of your life – of your relationship. But it's short-lived. Knowing that 'this too shall pass' is a mantra to repeat often. To be mentally tough, you have to have the will to push through difficulties.

4. Adaptability/Flexible Mindset
   Every animal and plant on earth has had to adapt in some way to survive. The ones that could not adapt to a changing environment died out. The ones that could change and evolve have survived. You must be able to adapt to a huge change in your life, sleeping patterns, your time. You must also be able to recognize the things that are worth continuing and the things that need to be abandoned. In a hurricane, a rigid tree resists the wind for a while but eventually gets blown over, while the flexible tree is more flexible and is able to bend with the wind and lives to face another storm.

"A newborn baby has only three demands. They are warmth in the arms of its mother, food from her breasts, and security in the knowledge of her presence. Breastfeeding satisfies all three."
–Grantly Dick-Read–

BREASTFEEDING—STARTING OUT RIGHT - DR. JACK NEWMAN

Breastfeeding is the natural, physiologic way of feeding infants and young children, and human milk is the milk made specifically for human infants. Formulas made from cow's milk or soybeans (most formulas, even "designer formulas") are only superficially similar, and advertising that states otherwise is misleading. Breastfeeding should be easy and trouble- free for most mothers. A good start helps to ensure that breastfeeding is a happy experience for both mother and baby.

The vast majority of mothers are perfectly capable of breastfeeding their babies. Read up on "laid-back breastfeeding" to see how easy breastfeeding can be. In fact, most mothers produce more than enough milk. Unfortunately, outdated hospital routines based on bottle feeding still predominate in too many health care institutions and make breastfeeding difficult, even impossible, for too many mothers and babies.

For breastfeeding to be well and properly established, a good start in the early few days can be crucial. Admittedly, even with a terrible start, many mothers and babies manage. The trick to breastfeeding is getting the baby to latch on well. A baby who latches on well gets milk well. A baby who latches on poorly has more difficulty getting milk, especially if the supply is low. A poor latch is similar to giving a baby a bottle with a nipple hole that is too small; the bottle is full of milk, but the baby will not get much.

When a baby is latching on poorly, he may also cause the nipple pain. And, if he does not get milk well, he will usually stay on the breast for long periods, thus aggravating the pain. Unfortunately, anyone can say that the baby is latched on well, even if he isn't. Too many people who should know better just don't know what a good latch is. Here are a few ways breastfeeding can be made easy:

A proper latch is crucial to success. Unfortunately, too many mothers are being "helped" by people who don't know what a proper latch is. If you are being told your two-day-old's latch is good despite your having very sore nipples, be skeptical, and ask for help from someone else who knows. Before you leave the hospital, you should be shown that your baby is latched on properly and that he is actually getting milk from the breast and that you know how to know he is getting milk from the breast (open mouth wide— pause— closed mouth type of suck). Look online for videos on how to latch a baby on (as well as other videos). If you and the baby are leaving the hospital not knowing this, get experienced help quickly (see handout *When Latching* on Dr. Newman's website). Some staff in the hospital will tell mothers that, if the breastfeeding is painful, the latch is not good (usually true) so the mother should take the baby off and latch him on again. This is not a good idea. The pain usually settles and the latch should be fixed on the other side or at the next feeding. Taking the baby off the breast and latching him on again and again only multiplies the pain and the damage.

The baby should be at the breast immediately after birth. The vast majority of newborns can be at the breast within minutes of birth. Indeed, research has shown that, given the chance, many babies only minutes old will crawl up to the breast from the mother's abdomen, latch on and start breastfeeding all by themselves. This process may take up to an hour or longer, but the mother and baby should be given this time together to start learning about each other. Babies who "self-attach" run into far fewer breastfeeding problems. This process does not take any effort on the mother's part, and the excuse that it cannot be done because the mother is tired after labor is nonsense, pure and simple. (Incidentally, studies have also shown that skin-to-skin contact between mothers and babies keeps the baby as warm as an incubator). Incidentally, many babies do not latch on and breastfeed during this time. Generally, this is not a problem, and there is no harm in waiting for the baby to start breastfeeding. The skin-to-skin contact is good for the baby and the mother even if the baby does not latch on.

The mother and baby should room in together. There is absolutely no medical reason for healthy mothers and babies to be separated from each other, even for short periods.

Health facilities that have routine separations of mothers and babies after birth are years behind the times and the reasons for the separation often have to do with letting parents know who is in control (the hospital) and who is not (the parents). Often, bogus reasons are given for separations. One example is that the baby passed meconium before birth. A baby who passes meconium and is fine a few minutes after birth will be fine and does not need to be in an incubator for several hours' "observation."

There is no evidence that mothers who are separated from their babies are better rested.

On the contrary, they are more rested and less stressed when they are with their babies. Mothers and babies learn how to sleep in the same rhythm.

Thus, when the baby starts waking for a feed, the mother is also starting to wake up naturally. This is not as tiring for the mother as being awakened from deep sleep, as she often is if the baby is elsewhere when he wakes up. If the mother is shown how to feed the baby while both are lying down side by side, the mother is better rested.

The baby shows long before he starts crying that he is ready to feed. His breathing may change, for example. Or he may start to stretch. The mother, being in light sleep, will awaken, her milk will start to flow and the calm baby will be content to nurse. A baby who has been crying for some time before being tried on the breast may refuse to take the breast even if he is ravenous.

Mothers and babies should be encouraged to sleep side by side in the hospital. This is a great way for mothers to rest while the baby nurses. Breastfeeding should be relaxing, not tiring.

Artificial nipples should not be given to the baby.

There seems to be some controversy about whether "nipple confusion" exists. Babies will take whatever gives them a rapid flow of fluid and may refuse others that do not.

Thus, in the first few days, when the mother is normally producing only a little milk (as nature intended), and the baby gets a bottle (as nature intended?) from which he gets rapid flow, the baby will tend to prefer the rapid flow method. You don't have to be a rocket scientist to figure that one out, though many health professionals, who are supposed to be helping you, don't seem to be able to manage it.

Note: It is not the baby who is confused. Nipple confusion includes a range of problems, including the baby not taking the breast as well as he could and thus not getting milk well and/or the mother getting sore nipples. Just because a baby will "take both" does not mean that the bottle is not having a negative effect. Since there are now alternatives available if the baby needs to be supplemented (see handout #5 on Jack Newman's website, *Using a Lactation Aid*, and handout #8, *Finger Feeding*), why use an artificial nipple?

No restriction on length or frequency of breast feedings. A baby who drinks well will not be on the breast for hours at a time. Thus, if he is, it is usually because he is not latching on well and not getting the milk that is available. Get help to fix the baby's latch, and use compression to give the baby more milk (handout #15, Breast Compression). Compression works very well in the first few days to get the colostrum flowing well

Supplements of water, sugar water, or formula are rarely needed. Most supplements could be avoided by getting the baby to take the breast properly and thus get the milk that is available. If you are being told you need to supplement without someone having observed you breastfeeding, ask for someone to help who knows what they are doing.

There are rare indications for supplementation, but often supplements are suggested for the convenience of the hospital staff. If supplements are required, they should be given by lactation aid at the breast (see handout #5), not cup, finger feeding, syringe or bottle. The best supplement is your own colostrum.

Free formula samples and formula company literature are not gifts. There is only one purpose for these "gifts" and that is to get you to use formula. It is very effective and it is unethical marketing. If you get any from any health professional, you should be wondering about his/her knowledge of breastfeeding and his/her commitment to breastfeeding. "But I need formula because the baby is not getting enough!" Maybe, but, more likely, you weren't given good help and the baby is simply not getting the milk that is available.

Even if you need formula, nobody should be suggesting a particular brand and giving you free samples. Get good help. Formula samples are not help.

Under some circumstances, it may be impossible to start breastfeeding early. However, most "medical reasons" (maternal medication, for example) are not true reasons for stopping or delaying breastfeeding, and you are getting misinformation. Get good help. Premature babies can start breastfeeding much, much earlier than they do in many health facilities.

In fact, studies are now quite definite that it is less stressful for a premature baby to breastfeed than to bottle-feed. Unfortunately, too many health professionals dealing with premature babies do not seem to be aware of this.

▌MINDFUL MOTHERING

You'll spend quite a bit of time sitting on the couch feeding your baby in the first few days. Netflix and chill will take on an entirely new meaning. You could use some of this time to catch up on Facebook or watch TV or you could use this time to be present with your baby. Eating is a social activity - imagine being out having lunch with a good friend and she spends the time checking her phone instead of connecting with you. I struggled with this in the early days of my baby moon with my son Cooper. Cooper was a frequent feeder and I found myself becoming frustrated with not being able to complete simple tasks such as emptying the dishwasher or finishing an email. As I sat "under" (rather than with) my beautiful boy, my mind raced to what I "needed" to do next and focused on all the things I wasn't getting done instead of paying more attention to my son and enjoying this short-lived time. It took me a few weeks to appreciate that I was doing something incredible, something much more worthwhile and important than emptying the dishwasher or ticking off the long checklist of to-dos." I was mothering my son and learning to do so mindfully, moment by moment, feed by feed. When I accepted that this was a 'season' in my life and things are always changing it became easier to accept what was happening with a lot more patience for myself and for my gorgeous boy who is now running off to play basketball with his friends.

As you feed your baby, try to be present on purpose, notice his soft skin, how he looks up at you, tune in to your baby's breathing and your own. Even just a couple of moments is a great start.

Can you be mindful and change a poopy diaper - absolutely! Notice your emotion ... are you exasperated with the millionth change today how does your body feel? Are you on autopilot and your mind is a million miles away? Can you be present on purpose for one or two diaper changes today?

"The biggest thing I remember is that there was just no transition. You hit the ground diapering."
–Paul Reiser–

CALMING YOUR BABY - WITH THE CUDDLE CURE

Most expectant couples will spend countless hours in prenatal classes learning all about birth: There's the yoga class, the breastfeeding class, and then newborn basics. By the time they get to their due date, most of them are just ready to get the show on the road, give up all these classes, and get on with the real business of having their baby. But, as more seasoned parents will tell you, it's only after birth that the real "labor" starts. You've probably seen that all-knowing smug smile creep across your mother-in-law's face when you tell her how tired you and your partner are from a day of shopping for the nursery. You probably only figured out what that look meant six months after your baby was born and maybe just reading this article right now you're having an Oprah "aha" moment and realizing exactly what she was so smug about.

Thankfully for first-time parents, changing a diaper and giving your baby a bath come relatively easily once someone has shown you how. But, with so many families spread all over the world, many new parents haven't even held a newborn before we held our own. As for calming a crying baby - well, for the uninitiated, it's not as easy as it looks. We've come to believe that it's our fate and even a parenting rite of passage that we have to endure hours of endless crying.

Not anymore, according to Dr. Harvey Karp, whose method of calming the fussiest babies has attracted worldwide attention. This is one lesson that you don't want to skip.

WHY DO BABIES CRY?

Babies cry for more reasons than I can include here. It's their way of communicating. It's essentially a survival mechanism. The most common reasons are that they are hungry, wet, tired, sick, or they just need a cuddle. In 1962, Dr. T. Berry Brazelton asked 82 new mothers to record how much their normal healthy babies cried each day during the first three months of life. (It's not clear from Dr. Brazelton's study if 'crying it out' was followed by these moms during the early 1960s.)

Dr. Brazelton discovered that, at two weeks of age, 25% of the babies cried for more than two hours each day. By six weeks, 25% cried for more than three hours a day. Reassuringly, he found that by three months almost all were back to crying for about one hour a day. Sometimes your baby may be diagnosed with "colic." A colicky baby will easily fit the following "profile": He will cry for three hours a day (usually evening) three days a week three weeks in a row.

While many experts have tried to find a pattern to this problem, there are no consistent links between a baby's gender, prematurity, or the baby's food. There are lots of theories about why some babies tend to be more colicky than others but none really hold true when investigated thoroughly. Most parents of colicky babies share similar experiences of their infants writhing and grunting, not being comforted by feeding or holding, they have a piercing cry like their baby is in severe pain.

IS IT COLIC?

Babies experiencing colic tend to be more fussy in the evenings and are inconsolable for hours which of course is very distressing for parents however not all cultures experience colic. In recent studies on crying patterns in newborns colic was found to be the highest in newborns in the UK (28% of newborns at 1–2 weeks), Canada (34.1% at 3–4 weeks), and Italy (20.9% at 8–9 weeks of age). The lowest figures were found in Denmark (5.5% at 3–4 weeks) and Germany (6.7% at 3–4 weeks).

Moms with a history of migraine are more likely to have a baby with colic but it's important to remember that colic is a time-limited phenomenon that generally resolves itself in a few weeks. Other factors that increase the risk of colic in newborns is maternal anxiety, post partum depression, low social support and even those gut microbes.

What you can do:

Get support – talk to other parents with similar experiences and be gentle with yourself. Always respond to your baby's cries as it's critical for his brain health but if you feel you cannot cope ask for help.

Wear baby in a sling – the movement and reassurance of your heartbeat and voice will help buffer your baby from excessive distress. Your ability to remain calm and compassionate helps your baby.

Dim the lights and note any strong smells that might be triggering the colic (especially due to the association with migraine).

Take a warm bath with your baby.

Over the counter gas relief drops have not been shown to resolve colic any better than placebo.

"You don't take a class; you're thrown into motherhood and learn from experience"
–Jennie Finch–

HAS DR. KARP FOUND THE HOLY GRAIL OF NEWBORN PARENTING?

The piercing cry of a baby immediately puts the mother and father's nervous systems on red alert. Your baby's cry is unique to your baby and was designed by nature to get your attention fast. When our ancestors lived in caves a baby left crying would attract wild animals. Moms are often reassured that they will eventually figure out what each "cry" means, but that's little comfort to a new mom and dad with a screaming infant on their hands after a long day at work - and for the first few weeks they all do sound the same. Or no doubt someone has told you not to pick up your baby each time he cries or you'll spoil him. You can't spoil a baby! Ignoring a baby and letting him "cry it out" would be like leaving your car alarm screeching until the battery eventually dies. Your baby does not have the brain capacity to manipulate you but parents have the capacity to damage their baby's brain by leaving their baby in a state of high distress. Trust your instincts and pick up your baby. Wearing your baby in a sling can make those first few weeks a lot more enjoyable for you and your baby.

A baby's cry is like a fire alarm going off...... and just as with a fire alarm, you don't know if it's your house burning or your toast.... just as your baby may only need to have a diaper change or he may need medical attention.

EASY WAYS TO CALM YOUR BABY - AKA THE CUDDLE CURE

Dr. Harvey Karp is a pediatrician and a child development specialist in Santa Monica, CA. He is also an assistant professor at the School of Medicine, UCLA. In the past 20 years of working with babies, Dr. Karp has taken the world of pediatrics by storm. Dr. Harvey Karp has spent many years trying to figure out the mystery of colic and why it affects some babies and not others. Through his research, he has developed an easy technique to turn even the fussiest baby into what he calls "The Happiest Baby on the Block." Like all of these strategies – see what works for you. My husband and I found swaddling and gentle shushing to work really well to settle our boys.

His highly successful method is based on four revolutionary concepts:

1. The Fourth Trimester: How to re-create the womblike atmosphere your newborn misses outside the womb by swaddling your baby.
2. The Calming Reflex: An "off switch" all babies are born with that quickly soothes crying.
3. The five S's: Five easy methods to turn on your baby's calming reflex.
4. The Cuddle Cure: How to combine the five S's to calm even the most colicky baby.

THE FIVE S'S DONE IN ORDER

Swaddling - Tight swaddling gives your baby the continuous touching and support your baby experienced while still in your womb. Other cultures have been doing this for centuries and "wear" their babies close to them. Interestingly, these same cultures don't have colic.

You've probably heard about weighted blankets and how they act as fabric 'hug machines' stimulating relaxation and reducing anxiety – it's thought that a swaddle works in the same way. Not all experts are in agreement when it comes to swaddling, so be sure to join the GentleBirth Mom's group on Facebook to keep up with the latest research recommendations.

Side/stomach position - You place your baby, while holding her, either on her left side to assist in digestion, or on her stomach to provide reassuring support. Once your baby is happily asleep, you can safely put her in her crib, on her back. Always place your baby on her back when sleeping to reduce the risk of SIDS.

Shushing Sounds - These sounds imitate the continual whooshing sound made by the blood flowing through arteries near the womb. Did you know the noise level that your baby is used to in the womb is equivalent to a loud vacuum cleaner? The good news is that you don't have to ruin your appliances by running the vacuum all day; instead, get a white noise App or MP3 that can be played over and over again. Babies are used to noise, so trying to soundproof his room to the noises of daily life (which he's used to listening to, anyway) will just stress you out even more.

Swinging - Newborns are used to the swinging, jiggling motions that were present when they were still in your womb. Every step you took, every movement caused a swinging motion for your baby (like that relaxing rocking sensation on a train). After your baby is born, this calming motion, which was so comforting and familiar, is abruptly gone. Your baby misses the motion and has a difficult time getting used to it not being there. Using a sling is ideal.

Sucking - "Sucking has its effects deep within the nervous system," notes Karp, "and triggers the calming reflex and releases natural chemicals within the brain." This "S" can be accomplished easiest with the breast, but a bottle or soother or even a finger will work too.

Not every baby will need all five techniques and, if you're breastfeeding, I would encourage you to offer the breast first. Calmer babies will need only a few, while fussier babies will need all of them. Gauge your success in calming your little one according to your baby's intensity. Like any other skill, it takes practice. My husband and I practiced swaddling on a stuffed toy and had it down to a fine art by the time my firstborn, Jack, arrived. Dr. Karp's Cuddle Cure may help make those first few weeks of new parenthood enjoyable instead of spending it desperately waiting to see that light at the end of the tunnel that everyone keeps talking about while you wish away those first fantastic weeks with your newborn.

ADJUSTING TO LIFE WITH YOUR NEWBORN

"Sometimes when you pick up your child you can feel the map of your own bones beneath your hands, or smell the scent of your skin in the nape of his neck. This is the most extraordinary thing about motherhood – finding a piece of yourself separate and apart that all the same you could not live without."
–Jodi Picoult–

If you're finding things challenging you might be thinking that there is a conspiracy of silence around parenthood. In the haze of pregnancy bliss, you didn't remember anyone telling you how exhausting those first few months can be or the brain fog that descends on you for weeks after your baby arrives and even remembering your name becomes difficult.

The midwife never mentioned the anxiety that comes with the realization that you are responsible for keeping this tiny being alive

24/7. There was definitely no mention of the F5 tornado that can descend on your relationship with the arrival of a newborn baby. Somebody definitely moved the goalposts.

Trust me – we did try to warn you in subtle and not so subtle ways – "Enjoy your sleep while you can," "Watch the whole season of This is Us in one day," etc. You thought to yourself "How hard can it be – babies are tiny and all they do is eat and sleep – I've got this."

So why is it that so many women feel duped after their much-awaited newborn comes along and reality sets in or is it that society has set us up to feel like we're 'failing' as mothers before we even begin. Part of the problem is that nothing prepares you for the first couple of weeks as a new mom. Not the 20 books from Amazon, not the daily updates from BabyCenter. It is what I like to call a 'lived' experience. Some moms adjust to life with a new baby so easily and others find it a more challenging transition (being very politically correct here). Breastfeeding puns aside those early weeks can sometimes really suck and it's ok to feel that way. But what's not ok is your evil twin having lots to say about your parenting abilities especially when you're already just trying to physically recover from birth. Remember more than ever in these early weeks – thoughts are not facts.

If you're finding things tough right now, know that you are not alone. The mom with the full makeup running with the Phil and Ted is probably just out the other end of three weeks of teething and a bout of mastitis. No matter how great she looks today or how well she seems to be adjusting, go sit down with a pot of coffee and a plate of brownies and you'll hear the universal story of mothers feeling like they are just winging it pretty much every day in the beginning.

Let's be honest society doesn't exactly cherish its new mothers the same way it cherishes that gorgeous new baby, but both need lots of TLC, support, and reassurance in those early weeks. Instead, we're sent packing from the hospital sometimes within hours of giving birth with no safety net for most and it's sink or swim.

A childless co-worker asks why you're so tired from 'just' being home all day with a baby – "how hard can that be?" she asks (no doubt with visions of you binge watching Netflix while baby sleeps peacefully for hours). You wonder if maybe you're not coping as well as everyone else seems to be and the doubt grows but before you entertain any notions of how others think early motherhood should be, consider this....

Consider how much endless patience and skill it takes to soothe a colicky baby who cries for hours on end.

Consider how much devotion it takes to care for every need of a newborn baby 24 hours a day. (The mom 'shift' never ends – sure, your partner might take over for a few hours when he gets in from work but mom brain never really clocks out).

Consider how much mental toughness is required to sit through Peppa Pig – again!

Consider how, in the words of Bruno Mars, you could love this tiny person so completely and deeply that you would literally catch a grenade for him.

Nobody warns you about the boredom and the loneliness. I make no apologies for stating that babies aren't exactly the most riveting conversationalists, particularly if you've been used to engaging in adult conversation for several hours a day in your professional life. They don't seem to do a lot of anything in the beginning but their brains are growing at warp speed and engaging with you throughout the day which makes all of that happen. Tell him about the weather, the food you're cooking, sing some Adele for him – your baby will adore it and making eye contact with your baby synchs up your brainwaves with his. These seemingly simple interactions grow your baby's brain at warp speed.

As one mother to another, I applaud you! So you didn't get the dishwasher emptied today and the pile of laundry is growing but what you did was nothing short of extraordinary – you mothered a newborn baby ALL day! You have my admiration, because between blowouts (not the hair styling kind) and Barney you are shaping the future of our society – one diaper change at a time. It is also perfectly okay to NOT love being a mom every minute of every day (some days you might not even like it and that's okay too).

In my eyes (and your baby's) you are a Superhero. Props to you.

If you feel you're not enjoying your baby as much as you think you should, here are a few ways to help you adjust to the changes.

Create a flexible routine for yourself – before you went on maternity leave you had a structured day – do the same now so you have simple achievable goals. If it all goes belly up because your baby is going through a growth spurt start again tomorrow.

Try to notice the snarky opinion of your evil twin, it means well but it's putting a huge downer on this special time in your life especially when it keeps comparing you to other moms who seem to have it all together. Your evil twin can spark postpartum depression and anxiety so listen closely to what it's saying and disregard anything that makes you feel bad.

Join a mom and baby group – you'll meet lifelong friends who are winging it just like you are – the honesty is so reassuring.

Outsource as much as you can (e.g. get a cleaner if you can afford it and, if not, then drop your standards a little and embrace the mess). Hire a postpartum doula to help you and your partner in those first few weeks.

Use technology to connect with other moms online especially in the winter and keep up your GentleBirth App (here's a secret...the App can be even more helpful for life AFTER birth).

Find easy ways to fill your cup, make some scheduled 'me time' a priority – even if it's just an undisturbed hour in the bath. (As a new parent sometimes even a trip to the supermarket alone can be replenishing!).

Talk to your care provider or a good friend if you're struggling.

*"I don't remember who said this,
but there really are places in the heart you
don't even know exist until you love a child."*
–Anne Lamott–

▌SWIMMING UPSTREAM

"When I think back to my own mom, she always seemed so on top of things. I feel dismayed and guilty that I'm not handling things as well and feel a lot more frazzled than she seemed to be."

Let's step back for a minute and look at how we got here. During more than 99% of the time that humans (or our close ancestors) have lived on this planet, mothers raised families in small groups of hunter-gatherers. If you had been among them, your life would have moved at the speed of a walk while you provided for your needs and fulfilled your ambitions with a child on your hip or nearby. You would have eaten fresh and organic foods saturated in micro-nutrients and you would have breathed air and drunk water free of artificial chemicals. Most important of all, you would have spent much of your day with other mothers, surrounded by a supportive community of relatives, friends, and neighbors. These are the conditions to which your body and mind are adapted for raising children. Nonetheless, at odds with this basic genetic blueprint, most mothers today must rush about stressfully, constantly juggling and multitasking. Few modern jobs can be done with young children around, so working means spending much of the day separated from your kids and the stresses of the unnatural schedule and pace they must then handle affect them in ways that naturally spill over onto you.

Unfortunately, while the essential activities of mothering - pregnancy, childbirth, breastfeeding, worrying and planning and loving with all your heart - have not altered one bit, our world has changed profoundly, and evolution hasn't had time to catch up. You and we are genetically identical to the first modern humans of 200,000 years ago, and nearly identical to our earliest tool-using ancestors, who lived over two million years ago.

Compared to our ancestors, most of us eat much fewer vegetables and whole foods, and much more white flour, sugar, and artificial chemicals, and we can't help absorbing some of the billions of pounds of toxins released into the environment each year, which even leave traces in breast milk. The so-called village it takes to raise a child usually looks more like a ghost town, so you have to rely more on your mate than did mothers in times past; but he, too, is strained by the unprecedented busyness and intensity of modern life.

If you feel like you're swimming upstream, it's because raising children was not meant to be this way. Many of the problems that seem purely personal or marital actually start on the other side of your front door.

Of course, the world is not going to change back to the time of the hunter-gatherers (and we'd miss refrigerators and telephones too much if it did!). And those times certainly had their own difficulties, such as famine and disease. But, like every mother, you can't help but feel the impact of the whirlwind we're all living in.

That's why we think it's so important for you and every mother to take active steps to lower her stresses and increase her resources: That's mother nurture.

Adapted from *Mother Nurture: A Mother's Guide to Health in Body, Mind, and Intimate Relationships,* by Rick Hanson, Ph.D., Jan Hanson, L.Ac., and Ricki Pollycove, M.D.

www.RickHanson.net

"Being a mom has made me so tired. And so happy."
–Tina Fey–

WHAT TENNIS CAN TEACH US ABOUT NEWBORN MENTAL HEALTH

"You'll spoil the baby"…"You're making a rod for your back" … "You'll never get him into his own bed" … "Don't pick him up every time he cries" …

"He can't possibly be hungry again" … "You need to toughen him up" … Does any of this sound familiar – if not – it will.

What is a new mom to do when this is the advice you're getting from well-meaning family and friends (and sometimes health care professionals) but, when you follow the advice, it feels so wrong And maybe you persevere and ignore your gut feeling because you believe everyone else knows more about this whole 'mothering' thing than you, especially when it's your first baby. I hope the information I'm going to share with you will reassure you that following your instincts and responding to your baby is not only good for your baby's mental health, it's good for yours too. Recordings of inconsolable babies crying are used in military torture, which is why it also feels like torture to you.

Imagine your baby's brain is like a Matryoshka doll. It is built from the bottom up...(imagine the tiny doll in the center)...followed by a bigger doll and another.....That's how your baby's brain develops. Like building a house, everything is connected but you have to put in a strong foundation first. The basic brain circuits your baby is born with are very simple but have two important functions – to let mom know "Hey, I need you right now....I'm hungry....I'm wet...I'm scared...I don't know what I need but I know I need you right now" so you will respond and help your baby grow the more complex areas of the brain needed to function as a healthy adult. So you've changed his nappy, and you know he's not hungry and your baby is still upset – and, again, well-meaning friends will say he's crying for 'no reason' ....or she's trying to manipulate you. Please understand that the world is a very big scary place for your baby and having you close by acts as a buffer to the stress of this scary world that your baby is constantly adjusting to.

Think of your relationship with your baby like a tennis match. You 'serve' and baby 'returns'....there's a constant 'to and fro' of communication. In the early days, that could simply be making eye contact, touching your baby, carrying your baby...cooing and talking to your baby and answering his cries. No Baby Einstein shows required!

As a new mom, it may seem like you're learning a new language but you're learning what your baby is communicating (as your brain is changing too).

Like a tennis match, every time your baby communicates to you through cries and body movement (that's the serve) and you respond appropriately consistently (return) you are growing your baby's brain in the healthiest way possible. Likewise, when you communicate with your baby and he responds, your brain is changing too! Win-win for you both!

As your baby gets older, you'll get lots of advice from other parents about sleep training or controlled crying but keep in mind your baby can only learn to comfort himself when your baby feels safe and secure – knowing his caregiver will respond to his needs. Not responding to your newborn baby's needs consistently (consistency is key) means his brain develops differently due to his ongoing stress response, so the growth in areas associated with regulating emotions and making decisions is smaller and the area associated with stress grows more. Being consistent is the key – don't feel guilty because your baby had to cry for a few minutes while you had the quickest shower of your life. So why is this important? Research suggests that adults with smaller executive functioning areas and smaller hippocampi tend to experience more physical and psychological complications in life (it's hard to make good decisions about your health or lifestyle when that part of the brain hasn't developed properly). Your baby is learning the capacity to trust. Right from those first moments after birth, your baby's brain is wired to build a relationship with you so he can survive and thrive.

Being a new mom can be incredibly hard and, if you have a colicky baby, it can test even the most patient parents...your baby is inconsolable and cries and cries...you've tried everything. Yes, this is a very stressful time for your baby (and parents) but, by doing everything you're already doing – walking, carrying baby in a sling, rocking etc and reacting calmly to your baby's distress, you are buffering that stress response in his brain. It might feel like what you're doing isn't helping but responding gently and compassionately is exactly what he needs right now while he goes through this tough time.

Your body has been your baby's habitat for the nine months of pregnancy and your body remains your baby's habitat (skin-to-skin on your chest) for the next few days after birth (or longer) as this magical brain wiring begins. Your baby's brain forms 700 – 1000 new neural connections every second of every day for the first two years of life and you are the person best equipped to help those connections happen in all the right places just by responding to your baby when he needs you.

So today respond gently to your baby, rock them to sleep in your tired arms one more time tonight grateful knowing that you are the expert on your baby and your instincts won't let you down. Lean on your family and friends for support on those difficult days so you're also not just surviving new motherhood but thriving too.

I Am Enough

GETTING YOUR GROOVE BACK

Sex and the New Mother

(an excerpt from BabyLune.com)

I know it's ridiculous, but my six-month-old still doesn't sleep through the night. She still wakes up for one nursing session. It wouldn't be so bad if I took naps or slept in, but I work these days and napping is not a possibility. My tiredness is having its effect on marital relations.

On Thursday, I thought my libido had come back. So, I thought I would sit beside my husband on the couch while he watched the World Cup and let nature take its course at half-time.

Then, I saw my freshly made bed with crisp, clean sheets, plump, soft pillows and cozy duvet. Pardon the clichés, but my bed is a conventional beauty. And king-sized.

It was only slightly dark in the early evening, but there was a slight breeze coming through the open window that made getting under the blankets just so inviting. To sleep.

I don't think my husband noticed I was gone!

SEX AFTER PREGNANCY: LET YOUR BODY SET THE PACE

After childbirth, sex may be the last thing on your mind. If you're feeling up to it, follow your sex drive where it leads.

Sex after pregnancy happens. Honestly. But first, vaginal soreness and sheer exhaustion are likely to take a toll. Whether you're in the mood or sex is the last thing on your mind, here's what you need to know about sex after pregnancy.

AFTER OUR BABY IS BORN, HOW SOON CAN I HAVE SEX?

Whether you give birth vaginally or by cesarean, your body will need time to heal. Many health care providers recommend waiting six weeks before resuming intercourse. This allows time for the cervix to close, postpartum bleeding to stop, and any tears or repaired lacerations to heal.

But the other important timeline is your own. Some women feel ready to resume sex within a few weeks of giving birth. Others need more time. Factors such as fatigue, postpartum blues, and changes in body image may take a toll on your sex drive.

WILL IT HURT?

Your vagina may be dry and tender, especially if you're breastfeeding. To ease any discomfort, take it slow. Start with cuddling, kissing, or massage. Gradually build the intensity of stimulation. If vaginal dryness is a problem, use a lubricating cream or gel. Try different positions to take pressure off any sore areas and control penetration. Tell your partner what feels good—and what doesn't. If sex continues to be painful, consult your doctor. Rarely, complications of healing may require additional treatment.

WILL IT FEEL DIFFERENT?

After several vaginal deliveries, decreased muscle tone in the vagina may reduce pleasurable friction during sex, which can influence arousal. To tone your pelvic floor muscles, remember to do your Kegel exercises and practice your perineal massage in pregnancy. (Encourage your partner to read this section as an incentive for him to help you with your GentleBirth practice). I recommend all moms see a women's pelvic health wellness physiotherapist 6 weeks after birth whether you had a vaginal or cesarean birth. Too many moms are suffering from painful sex and urinary incontinence months after birth.

WHAT ABOUT BIRTH CONTROL?

Unless you're hoping to become pregnant right away, sex after pregnancy requires a reliable method of birth control even if you're breastfeeding. Barrier methods such as condoms and spermicides can be useful. If you prefer hormonal birth control, it's important to select a method that doesn't interfere with breastfeeding. Your postpartum checkup is a great time to ask your midwife or obstetrician about the options.

WHAT IF I'M TOO TIRED TO HAVE SEX?

Caring for a newborn can be exhausting. If you're too tired to have sex at bedtime, say so. But that doesn't mean your sex life is over. You may prefer making love early in the morning or during your baby's nap. Feed your baby first to extend the time you and your partner have together.

WHAT IF I'M NOT INTERESTED IN SEX?

That's okay. There's more to a sexual relationship than intercourse, especially when you're adjusting to life with a new baby. If you're not feeling sexy or you're afraid sex will hurt, share your concerns with your partner. Until you're ready to have sex, maintain intimacy in other ways. Spend time together without the baby, even if it's just a few minutes in the morning and after the baby goes to sleep at night. Share short phone calls throughout the day or occasional soaks in the tub. Look for other ways to express affection.

If communicating with your partner doesn't help, be alert for signs and symptoms of postpartum depression. If your mood is consistently low, you find little joy in life, or you have trouble summoning the energy to start a new day, contact your doctor promptly.

WHAT CAN I DO TO BOOST MY SEX DRIVE?

Go easy on yourself. The thing is it's hard to get in the mood with your evil twin insisting you are so unattractive to your partner these days and repeatedly harping on about losing the baby weight. She will play on every insecurity and vulnerability you thought you left behind with your teenage years – and she is MEAN!

Set reasonable expectations as you adjust to life with your new baby. Appreciate the changes in your body. Eat healthy foods, and drink plenty of fluids. Try to get in some exercise. Make 'me' time a priority. Self-care goes a long way toward keeping passion alive.

"There is only one pretty child in the world and every mother has it."
–Chinese Proverb–

EMOTIONAL HEALTH BEFORE AND AFTER YOUR BABY ARRIVES

Thankfully, postnatal (and prenatal) depression is starting to be discussed more openly. Most moms adjust well to the new world order and don't get depressed. It's estimated that around 10 to 20% of moms will experience postnatal depression (PND) and nearly 70% get well with low intervention (in most cases, medication isn't necessary). Self-help strategies such as CBT are considered among the most effective therapies for moms with mild to moderate depression (A grade therapy). Women who practice mindfulness tend to experience lower rates of anxiety and postpartum depression.

The realities of parenthood can be a shock to the system, especially for some older moms with established careers. If you're feeling low, there's a good chance that you're not depressed but may be experiencing anemia, an infection after birth, or thyroid problems. Maybe you're experiencing relationship problems or not getting any sleep.

Most moms experience the hormonal free-fall of the "baby blues" in the first few days after birth, but this is a hormonal reaction and resolves itself quickly.

Here are some helpful ways to help you assess if you may be suffering from depression or anxiety during your pregnancy or postnatally.

- Overall, how are things?
- Are you enjoying your pregnancy? Are you enjoying your new baby?
- How are you adapting to your new life?
- Over the past two weeks, have you had any down days? Do you feel like you're having more bad days than good?

If you aren't enjoying your new baby as much as you should, with more bad days than good for two weeks or more, it may be time to get help. Untreated PND can impact your baby's brain development because moms experiencing PND often don't engage with their baby the way other moms do and dads can also become depressed. Don't wait. If you think you may be depressed, talk to your healthcare provider. The sooner you start, the sooner you can fully enjoy your pregnancy and this new phase of your life with your new baby.

So, as you approach the end of the program, you may still have some 'wobbles' toward the end of your pregnancy. This is totally normal. You are about to embark on the adventure of a lifetime and bring a new human into the world - it would be strange not to have any wobbles at all.

TOOLS FOR PARENTS – EDINBURGH POSTNATAL DEPRESSION SCREENING

There are some problems using EPDS as a screening tool that are common with any type of screening tool for PND:

- It doesn't necessarily pick up all symptoms, and it's less helpful if you are suffering from anxiety, but it is recognized as being a useful guide to how you are feeling at the time.
- The other difficulty with postnatal depression is that some days you might feel fine while other days are especially difficult.

The above can result in what are commonly called "false positive" or "false negative" results where the screening tool does not work. That is why EPDS is normally completed with the help of a trained health care professional who can provide a clinical diagnosis of anxiety, depression or PTSD for which they may use detailed questionnaires or assessment tools.

You might find it helpful to follow this link to take an online version of the Edinburgh Postnatal Depression quiz and follow up with your care provider.

https://healthyfamilies.beyondblue.org.au/

SAD DADS

As a new mom, you're carrying the bulk of this huge transition but remember that many new fathers are anxious and stressed about their new responsibilities as well and most don't talk about it. Just like you, they feel thrown in at the deep end and most dads feel unprepared for the realities of life with a newborn, little sleep and a partner who is recovering physically too. Most dads really want to be involved and provide you with meaningful support but that kind of dad 'training' isn't always easy to find (a great reason to come along to a GentleBirth workshop so you're both on the same page mentally and emotionally). When you combine uncertainty, stress, lack of sleep and the opinions of your combined evil twins, it can quickly lead to anxiety, which can put your partner on a fast track to depression.

Several studies have confirmed that mental health issues with new fathers constitute a growing concern. One European organization found that more than 1 in 3 new fathers (38%) are concerned about their mental health. Overall, the current research suggests that 1 in 10 dads have PND. Fathers also appear to be more likely to suffer from depression three to six months after their baby is born. Paternal depression is even more common (50%) when mom is experiencing mood concerns too. We know that postpartum depression in women is multifactorial and involves hormones, brain chemistry and the huge life adjustment that comes with being a new parent. Dads experience all of the above also but often with additional stressors such as being the sole breadwinner.

The stigma against experiencing difficulties in early parenthood is even higher for men than for women. We expect them to be stoic, strong and selfless but when a new dad is having difficulties they're even less likely to ask for help.

WHAT SYMPTOMS SHOULD PARTNERS LOOK OUT FOR AND WHERE CAN THEY GO FOR SUPPORT?

With normal stress partners will feel better after some extra sleep or meeting a friend or exercising but with depression, these things won't make him feel better and the symptoms are more severe and last longer. Ideally, dads should get help from a mental health professional who specializes in working with men as it's unlikely to improve and more likely to worsen without help.

PND affects each man differently but some of the more common signs are:

- Feeling very low over a 2 week period, often accompanied by feelings of hopelessness.
- Difficulty sleeping (not unusual for parents with a new baby but in this case your mind is racing and won't switch off).
- Withdrawing from the family (spending more time away from your partner and newborn).
- Feeling overwhelmed and wanting to cry or feelings of anger.
- Having disturbing thoughts about harming themselves or their baby.

Don't ignore it. This isn't something you can just 'get over' – it's a serious health condition that can also seriously impact your baby's development. A father's postpartum depression can have a negative and long-term impact on the psychological, social, and behavioral development of his children— even more so with baby boys regardless of whether the mom is depressed. If both parents are depressed, your child's development is even more severely impacted.

Talk to your partner. Speak to a care provider who can refer you to a specialist. We need to treat brain health the way we treat any other kind of health issue and talk about it the same way. There would be no shame in going to your GP because you had a knee injury or heart condition – brain health should be no different.

There is a silver lining – most parents with a diagnosis of mild to moderate depression will have a complete recovery and, more often than not these days, medication isn't the first recommended option for treatment.

> You're not alone, it's not your fault, you're not to blame.

Final words from Tracy

Forget YOLO (you only live once) and consider YOBO instead. You only get one chance to give birth to this baby - make it the best experience it can be for both of you. You've got this!

As you continue on your journey into motherhood enjoy this story...

Once upon a time, there was a bunch of tiny frogs... who arranged a running competition (yeah yeah I know frogs don't run...use your imagination).

The goal was to reach the top of a very high tower.

A big crowd had gathered around the tower to see the race and cheer on the contestants....

The race began....

Honestly, no one in the crowd really believed that the tiny frogs would reach the top of the tower.

You heard statements such as: "Oh, it's WAY too difficult!!" "They will NEVER make it to the top, they should just give up." The tiny frogs began collapsing, one by one....

Except for those, who in a fresh tempo, were climbing higher and higher....

The crowd continued to yell, "It is too difficult!!! No one will make it!" More tiny frogs got discouraged and tired and gave up ...

But ONE continued higher and higher and higher ... she just wouldn't give up.

At the end, everyone else had given up climbing the tower. Except for the one tiny frog who, remaining focused on the tower, was the only one who reached the top! All of the other tiny frogs naturally wanted to know how this one frog managed to do it? A contestant asked the tiny frog how he had found the strength to succeed and reach the goal.

It turned out ...

That the winner was deaf...

The wisdom of this story is that you should never listen to other people's tendencies to be negative or pessimistic ... because they take your most wonderful dreams and wishes away from you.

Always remember the power words have because everything you hear and read affects your beliefs.

So when anyone wants to tell you how difficult labor will be or how naïve you are - just pretend to be deaf!

Wishing you a wonderful birth and very positive parenting experience.

All is well.

Tracy Donegan

Registered Midwife

Instead of the usual "what ifs" we tend to hear about birth, consider the following very possible scenarios........

What If........

I have a wonderful calm gentle birth......
I really can do this......
I can handle anything that comes my way......
I'm stronger than I realize......
I give birth calmly, with confidence and in control......
I give birth without fear......
I nurse my baby easily......
I love being a mom and enjoy this new season of my life......

EPIDURAL PREFERENCES

Thank you for your support on this special day and your help in avoiding potential nerve/pelvic organ/pelvic floor injury from common practices used with an epidural. My partner (and doula) will remain with me in the room while the epidural is being administered for emotional support.

I will be using the GentleBirth App during and after the administration of the epidural to help me remain calm and still during the procedure.

Labor

Please provide me with a peanut ball and allow for frequent position changes during the first stage of labor. I may request that the epidural infusion is turned down to allow for more effective pushing.

As long as my baby and I are well I prefer to labor down and not start any active pushing until my baby is at +2 station to reduce exhaustion unless I have a strong urge before then.

I prefer a mother led non coached 2nd stage if I can feel the urge to push.

If I have adequate control of my legs I would like to try various positions including hands and knees. My partner and doula will assist.

If available please provide a squat bar to assist in my pushing efforts in an upright position to avoid being on my back.

**To create more space for my baby my ankles need to be further apart than my knees for internal rotation of my femur bones. If my knees are further apart than my feet the space at the pelvic outlet is reduced.

**In the event stirrups are necessary please move my legs simultaneously with another staff member or my partner when lifting in and out of stirrups. Please keep in mind the position of my ankles to create more space.

To reduce the risk of back/pelvic injury please to not direct me to pull my legs back or for my partner to push my head forward.

I prefer no vaginal stretching or massaging of my perineum.

Please do not use mineral oil, baby shampoo or any lubricant on my perineum.

When my baby's head is visible please apply a warm compress to my perineum to reduce the risk of perineal trauma. I am aware that I will be unable to gauge the temperature of the compress so please test it on my arm first.

I do not consent to an episiotomy without briefly discussing the medical necessity first.

I would appreciate your expert guidance to focus as my baby's head crowns.

Please do not suction my baby on the perineum routinely.

Assisted Birth

If instruments are required to assist my baby and a vacuum is being considered I understand an episiotomy is unlikely to be necessary.

If a forceps is advised I would like the most senior Obstetrician to perform the procedure.

To be discussed prenatally with staff.

If a forceps is recommended and there is time I would prefer that my baby is born by cesarean birth.

Suturing

Please ensure I have adequate analgesia for any suturing that may be needed and keep me covered until suturing is about to begin and Please only place my legs in stirrups right before suturing is about to begin to avoid the risk of blood clots.

Thank you for your support on this special day.

RECOMMENDED READING

Mindful Pregnancy (2020) by Tracy Donegan

The Irish Better Birth Book by Tracy Donegan

The Irish Cesarean and VBAC Guide by Tracy Donegan

Ina May Gaskin's Guide to Childbirth by Ina May Gaskin

Mother Nurture by Rick Hanson

Real Food for Pregnancy by Lily Nichols

What Mothers Do: Especially When It Seems Like Nothing by Naomi Stadlen

Mindful Motherhood by Cassandra Vieten

Made in the USA
Las Vegas, NV
08 February 2021